DEDICATION

To those who build on strengths:

My parents, George and Jeanne C. Tice
My aunt, Ethel W. Saulle
My friend, Colette Bernard
CJT

My brother, Dennis Dee Moore
Our mother, Mrs. M., and
The memory of our father, Wallace Moore
My beloved cousin, Hope Spitz
KP

About the Authors

Carolyn J. Tice Carolyn Tice, DSW, ACSW, is Associate Professor and Chair of the Department of Social Work at Ohio University, where she teaches courses in social welfare policy and mental health. For the last two years, she has been editor of AGENDA, a national newsletter on gerontology in social work education. Prior to teaching, Dr. Tice was director of media in social work education and practice. Her interests include the use of media in social work education and practice. Publications include "Supported Employment in Rural Environments: Implications for Social Work Practice" and "Using Films to Challenge Ageism."

Kathleen Perkins Kathleen Perkins, MSW, DSW, and MA in Social Gerontology, is Associate Professor, School of Social Work, at Louisiana State University. She worked as a research consultant with the Gray Panthers from 1986 to 1988 investigating retirement conditions of women in the Philadelphia metropolitan area and applied her findings to design pre-retirement planning programs for women. Dr. Perkins's expertise includes mental health issues for older adults. Publications include "Psychological Implications of Women and Retirement," "Recycling Poverty: From the Workplace to Retirement," and, co-authoring with Dr. Tice, "A Comparative Analysis of Long-term Care Policies and Services Between United States and Great Britain."

Contents

Preface

THIS BOOK DISCUSSES MENTAL HEALTH ISSUES of older adults and presents a strengths model practice for mental health and health care providers, such as social workers, counselors, clergy, nurses, nurse's aids, and physical and occupational therapists. The book is intended to be a professional handbook as well as a textbook for graduate and undergraduate education. The book's focus is timely for several reasons. First, America's population is aging at an unprecedented rate. Presently, one-quarter of the population is over the age of 75; by the year 2030, one-third of the population will be over 75 years old (Macaroy, 1991; Fowles, 1986). This demographic change suggests more support of aged individuals must be provided if they are to live decently and with respect. It is anticipated that many older people will become permanent patients in nursing homes or other protected settings. Some will have families, many will not.

Second, although the overall number of older adults is increasing, their use of mental health services has remained appreciably lower than their proportion in the general population. During the 1990s, an estimated 2% of older adults will receive services in psychiatric clinics and approximately 6% will be seen by community mental health practitioners (Kramer, Taube, & Redick, 1973; Edinburg, 1985; Butler, Lewis & Trey, 1991). Resources invested in services for people who are 65 years and older in some community mental health centers (CMHCs) are as low as 0 percent, and in 1990, 35% of CMHCs offered no specialized service for older adults (Speer, Williams, West, & Dupree, 1991).

Third, the underserving of older people is not indicative of their needs. Studies suggest that from 15 to 25% of the elderly population are faced with persistent mental health issues (Pfeiffer, 1977; Gurland & Toner, 1982; Kart, 1990). Blazer and Williams's (1980) findings suggested depressive symptomatology was present in 4 to 15% of older adults living in the community and 32 to 47% of older people residing in long-term care facilities. Further, the suicide rate for elderly individuals is about three times that of the general population (Edinburg, 1985).

A final reason that focus on mental health and the strengths model is timely is that older adults of today and tomorrow are and will be diverse racially, sexually, and ethnically. However, a common thread transcends this diversity: They are survivors. A strengths model for social work practice builds on that common thread by learning how people manage to live, perhaps thrive, in an often oppressive environment.

The book's purpose is to define and apply a strengths-based model of practice to mental health issues confronting older adults. The model departs from the traditional approaches by shifting from a pathology or problem orientation to an approach based on the strengths, past achievements, and interests of people. Further, the model emphasizes that assessment and service delivery involve a mutual enterprise between older people, their formal and informal support systems, and the social worker. This feature is essential for keeping individuals engaged, not only in the helping process, but in life in general.

The book's content is significant because it conveys expectations for change and outcomes. Additionally, the content encourages people to recognize and capitalize on their individual and joint power. Thus, a strengths model of practice is critical for the nation's older individuals, who, because of their stage in the life cycle, experience challenges in virtually every facet of their lives. Rather than labeling people according to their challenges or defining challenges as "problems" in an attempt to diagnose the needs of older adults, the book's conceptual framework encourages the identification, exploitation, and enhancement of the strengths that have assisted individuals to cope with and learn from complex realities throughout their lives.

Divided into three chapters, the book's first part moves from the philosophy and principles of the strengths perspective to a strengths model of practice and assessment. The second part discusses four mental health issues: depression, suicide, alcohol, and anxiety. These topics were selected because of their prevalence in older adults, their potential to lead to persistent mental conditions, and their disruptive social, emotional, and physical consequences for older adults, their families, and society as a whole.

The book's final section discusses the prevention of mental health disorders in older adults through social work practice based on strengths. This section recognizes that family dynamics and living situations of older people are not stagnant. In fact, life cycle issues and changing roles often force older adults to alter their perceptions and expectations of relationships, of care, and of their physical capabilities. To address the loss and stress often associated with aging, the strengths model presents adaptive and preventive strategies associated with retirement, long-term care, and the baby boom generation. The strengths perspective considers curative approaches to life-cycle events. The goal is guidelines for positive psychological and social preparation for later adulthood.

In conclusion, the book describes anticipated mental health needs of America's aging population and the responses of the mental health community. Recommendations for service providers, grounded in the strengths-based model, are offered in the form of action strategies. Such strategies consider the environment as a resource, review professional training, present research topics, and outline social policy initiatives.

The integrating theme of the book is the need to improve the availability and the quality of mental health services for older people. Such services should include an array of programs to address the wants of individuals with persistent mental challenges. Such services also include programs to enhance and nurture a person's mental health. Given the complex nature of the mental health system as it relates to older adults, a general approach to the topic is presented along with a comprehensive application of the strengths-based model for practice.

ACKNOWLEDGMENTS

This book represents a 3-year collaboration and the authors' interests in aging and social policies. Support for our early work came from Claire Verduin of Brooks/Cole and a grant from the Ohio University Resource Center.

Paul Pegher and Erin Spraw, two Ohio University students, provided me with technical assistance throughout the writing of this book. Their talents translated my ideas into many of the book's tables and figures. *CJT*

Many people have offered support throughout the writing of this book. I am deeply indebted to my friend and colleague Margaret Severson, who helped the manuscript along with her thoughtful suggestions and continual encouragement. Thanks goes to my graduate assistants, Yevette Robinson and Jackie Benoit, for their technical assistance on Chapters 4, 7, and 8.

I wish to warmly thank my friends from the Breakfast Club, as well as Mona Romaine, Marie Hoops, and my children, Tracie, Kelly, and Stephanie Perkins. They celebrated the birth of this book with me and boosted my spirits by asking for progress reports along the way.

I am especially indebted to Carlo Cuneo, a newfound friend, student, and colleague, who improved the manuscript with his careful line editing. *KP*

A number of reviewers read the manuscript, offering valuable suggestions and insights. We would like to thank Stephen Z. Cohen, University of Illinois at Chicago (retired); Dana Stuart Cole, Central Washington University; Enid Cox, University of Denver; Katherine Dunlap, University of North Carolina at Chapel Hill; Beverly C. Favre, Southern University at New Orleans; John B. Franz, California State University–Fresno; Anne-Linda Furstenberg, University of North Carolina at Chapel Hill; Christine Pollastro, Washington State University; Kathleen Reynolds, Madonna University; Margaret Severson, Louisiana State University.

Finally, we wish to express our thanks to Lisa Gebo, our current editor at Brooks/Cole, for her encouragement for the completion of this book.

REFERENCES

Blazer, D. & Williams, C. D. (1980). Epidemiology of dysphoria and depression in an elderly population. *American Journal of Psychiatry, 137,* 439–444.

Edinberg, M. (1985). *Mental health practice with the elderly.* Englewood Cliffs, NJ: Prentice-Hall.

Fowles, D. (Ed.). (1980). *Mental hygiene in the twentieth century.* New York: Arno Press.

Fowles, D. (1986). Discovering the older market. *Aging, 352,* 36–37.

Gurland, E., & Toner, J. A. (1982). Depression in the elderly: A review of recently published studies. In C. Eisdorfer (Ed.), *Annual review of geriatrics and gerontology* (pp. 228–265). New York: Springer Publishing Co.

Kart, C. S. (1990). *The realities of aging.* Boston: Allyn & Bacon.

Kramer, M., Taube, C. A., & Redick, R. W. (1973). Patterns of use of psychiatric facilities by the aged: Past, present, and future. In C. Eisdorfer & M. F. Lawton (Eds.), *Psychology of adult development and aging* (pp. 428–509). Washington, DC: American Psychological Association.

Macaroy, D. (1991). *Certain change.* Silver Spring, MD: National Association of Social Workers.

Pfeiffer, E. (1977). Psychopathy and social pathology. In J. Birren and K. Schaie (Eds.), *Handbook of the psychology of aging* (pp. 650–671). New York: Van Nostrand Reinhold Co.

Speer, D. C., Williams, J., West, H., & Dupree, L. (1991). Older adult users of outpatient mental health services. *Community Mental Health Journal, 27*(1), 69–75.

CHAPTER ONE

The Mental Health System and Older Adults

ALTHOUGH PROFESSIONAL, SOCIAL, cultural, and economic barriers limit exact definition of mental health and mental illness, there is general agreement that the terms represent opposite ends of a continuum (Mechanic, 1989). Individuals with persistent mental illness are often considered a danger to themselves or others and, because of their psychotic behavior, are perceived as being unable to function in community settings. As a result, they are frequently involuntarily placed in restrictive environments until their behavior becomes more compatible with the norms of the society.

In contrast, mental health connotes the ability to cope and accept the stresses associated with life. When faced with extraordinary circumstances, such as divorce, death, or illness, some people seek professional help in adjusting to the transitional period. Others depend on family and community support to regain a sense of balance. In either case, the ability to function in society is only minimally, if at all, interrupted, and an active, positive orientation to life is maintained.

Historical Overview

What role has the mental health system played in the lives of older adults? A brief historical perspective is necessary to gain an understanding of America's mental health system and policies in relation to the elderly.

Many of the current perceptions and attitudes toward mental health and mental illness originated in Europe and influenced developments in the United States. Foucault (1965) wrote that during the 1500s, as leprosy disappeared in Europe, insanity or madness emerged to symbolize the decay of mind and spirit. Insane individuals of any age were avoided and encouraged to wander the outer boundaries of towns and villages. If they became too numerous or troublesome, people with mental illness were transported to another location in "ships of fools" and left to wander again. Shunned by family members, church organizations, and the community, people unable to cope with these challenges were considered demonic and riddled with vice.

Approximately a century after the ships of fools stopped sailing, houses of confinement were constructed to shelter and isolate people perceived undesirable by society. Included in this category were people with mental illness. Within the houses of confinement, little in the way of treatment was provided. Rather, emphasis was on custodial care and strict work schedules to minimize the sin of idleness. Work was viewed as a solution to poverty of the mind and resources.

The idea of treatment for the mentally ill developed in 1792. The French physician Philippe Pinel introduced the concept of "moral treatment" and unchained the patients at Bicêtre, one of the two principal institutions in Paris for the mentally ill. The rubric of moral treatment assumed psychiatric illness could be alleviated by treating patients in a considerate and friendly fashion, providing them the opportunity to discuss their problems, stimulating their interests, and involving them in life activities. Mechanic (1989) stated the significance of moral treatment was its emphasis on medical personnel. A doctor played no part in houses of confinement. However, in the asylum and in the context of moral treatment, authority was vested in the physician far beyond the rudimentary knowledge medical personnel had of mental illness at the time.

Moral treatment was practiced in Massachusetts's Worcester State Hospital, established in 1830 as the first state hospital in the United States for the mentally ill. Hospital records indicate patients were offered humanistic care in an optimistic environment. Unfortunately, moral treatment did not persist. Grob (1966) concluded that for most of the nineteenth century the hospital was directed by pessimistic ideology. The societal influences that led to the deterioration of the hospital included industrial and technical changes, increased urbanization, and a growing number of patients. As the social value of mentally ill patients decreased with the rise of capitalism, their care became more restrictive and custodial in nature.

Given the increasingly offensive nature of institutions, the time was right for reform. In the mid-1800s, Dorothea Dix launched a successful national and international campaign to improve the quality of life within mental institutions. Through exhaustive documentation of on-site observations, she convinced state governments to repair, renovate, and rebuild institutions, integrate structured activities in the daily schedule of mental health patients, and insure a decrease in the mistreatment of individuals living in institutions. Initially, patients benefited from the additional physical and mental care, but the increasing number of people entering mental health institutions, followed by the subsequent growth in the size of institutions, significantly offset Dix's gains (DiNitto, 1991).

Following the reform work of Dorothea Dix, Clifford Beers directed public attention to the needs of people with mental illness in 1909 by forming the National Mental Health Association. His book, *A Mind That Found Itself* (1923) provided a vivid account of his two years as a mental patient, described the abusive environment typical of mental institutions at the time, and urged reforms in patient care. Beers's reform approach, referred to as the "mental hygiene movement," stimulated some improvements in the physical conditions of some institutions and increased public awareness of the needs of mentally ill patients (Grob, 1980). However, inadequate patient/staff ratios and untrained direct care workers minimized the efforts of Beers and supported the continuation of a custodial philosophy.

Current Mental Health Policy

The American mental health system and policies of today began to take shape in the aftermath of World War II as exemplified by the 1946 Mental Health Act. This legislation, which focused on training, education, and research, gained support during World War II when psychiatric screening was used to reject individuals from military service (DiNitto, 1991; Mechanic, 1989). The sheer number of people rejected for mental illness was enough to generate public support for social policy to address the diagnosis and treatment of mental illness. Although the legislation made no specific provisions for older people, it did make public the state of the nation's mental health and provided a background for future legislation.

In the 1950s, psychotherapeutic drugs dramatically changed mental health services. Drugs often reduced or controlled the symptoms of mental conditions, including auditory and visual hallucinations, suicidal ideation, and disorientation. Patients maintained on chemical regimes became more cooperative and receptive to treatment. In turn, patients and hospital personnel gained renewed confidence in community discharges. However, people did not receive adequate support from the mental health system (Rapp, 1992). As a result, 70% of people discharged were readmitted (Goldman, Adams, & Taube, 1983).

The Community Mental Health Act of 1963 began to address problems associated with community-based services by providing funds for the establishment and staffing of community mental health centers throughout the nation. Originally, the Act provided for five essential services: inpatient care, outpatient care, emergency care, partial hospitalization, and consultation and education (DiNitto, 1991).

In 1975, the Act was amended for the fifth time. This revision mandated special programs for individuals 65 years of age and older. This legislation marked the first time older adults were recognized as a group needing special attention by the mental health system. The amendment focused on aftercare services for those individuals with prior psychiatric admissions, halfway houses to facilitate the transfer from institutions to communities, and community-based screenings for individuals in need of mental health services.

A decade after the Older Americans Act of 1965, the 1975 amendments to the Community Mental Health Act, along with the Medicare provision of the Social Security Amendments of 1965, changed the availability of mental health services to older adults. Specifically, Medicare provided the financial vehicle for older adults to gain access to the mental health system. Unfortunately, financial backing has not been sufficient to break through the major barriers to providing mental health services to the elderly. Included in the barriers are cultural conflicts, lack of access to services, and overriding needs for basic resources such as food, shelter, and clothing (Edinberg, 1985).

In addition to service barriers, there is a strong possibility that stereotypes or myths negatively influence the participation of older adults in the mental health system. For example, Sue (1977) argued that mental health issues of older Asian-Americans are underestimated because providers stereotypically believe this group has no problems. Another myth is that older adults will not accept or trust the mental health practitioner (Edinberg, 1985). Although client distrust may be the case occasionally, the practitioner may set a cycle of self-fulfilling prophecy in motion by retaining a generalized expectation of distrust.

Perhaps one of the most pervasive barriers to delivering mental health services to older people is ageism, the "negative images of and attitudes toward people simply because they are old" (Zastrow, 1993, p. 461). Because ageism involves both prejudice and discrimination, its tentacles reach into virtually every aspect of life, including economic status, language, interpersonal relationships, and self-identity. Consequently, ageism must be confronted if the mental health system is to meet the wants and needs of older people. Ideally, ageism will be replaced by truths including (a) a decline in mental health is not inevitable in older adults, (b) older adults are not victims of senescence but survivors of life, and (c) the strengths of older people must be recognized, celebrated, and used as a cornerstone in intervention and prevention services.

Building on Strengths

Social work, much like other human services, unravels life's complexities by dividing issues into stark divisions between problem and solution, victim and villain, and deficit and strength. The origins of these dichotomies are found in the profession's history, which began with the concept of moral deficiency. The emphasis on individual deficits or frailties as the cause of difficulties is a theme that has continued in social work practice.

Although social work practice has a bias toward theoretical structures that define and label problems, the profession has not ignored the importance of building on individual and group strengths. The structure and principles of Perlman's (1957) problem-solving model presented a departure from Freudian-based psychodynamic "diagnostic" social work practice of diagnosing or labeling that emphasized pathology (Turner, 1986).

Functional theory, pioneered by Jessie Taft and Virginia Robinson of the School of Social Work at the University of Pennsylvania, highlighted the significance of client choice and self-determination (Robinson, 1930; Turner, 1986). Ruth Smalley (1967) applied functional theory to principles of practice based on purposive choices and decisions made by the person being helped. Bertha Reynolds (1951) suggested, "Our first question to the client should not be 'What problems bring you here today?' but rather, 'You have lived thus far, how have you done it?'" (p. 275). More recent writers, including Hepworth and Larsen (1990), Shulman (1979), and Germain and Gitterman (1980), have stressed the importance of expanding assessments to include a focus on individual strengths and included the client as an active participant in the change process.

Saleebey (1992) advanced the assessment of strengths by articulating a strengths perspective for social work practice. According to Saleebey, the strengths perspective is represented by a collation of ideas and techniques rather than theory or a paradigm. It "seeks to develop abilities and capabilities in clients" and "assumes that clients already have a number of competencies and resources that may improve their situation" (Saleebey, 1992, p. 15).

The philosophical differences between a problem-solving orientation and the strengths perspective are displayed in Table 1.1. The analysis highlights two central points. First, the assumptions of a problem orientation have contributed fundamental underpinnings for social work practice. When applying a problem orientation to practice,

TABLE 1.1 *Comparing Philosophical Frameworks:*
Problem Orientation and Strengths Perspective

	PROBLEM ORIENTATION	STRENGTHS PERSPECTIVE
Primary Emphasis	Assessing and addressing problems of deficits	Assessing and building on strengths
Nature of Intervention	Practitioner legitimizes course of action	Designed to maximize client self-direction
	Linear approach to alleviate symptoms of problem	Holistic approach to client's situation
	Services provided based on needs of clients	Services emphasize wants of clients
	Often limits clients to routine services	Maximizes collaborative efforts between client and informal and formal support systems
Orientation to Mental Health	Person Centered: Attempts to locate specific cause of the illness in the client	Ecological Approach: Recognizes multiple levels of influence internal and external to the client
Role of Client	Hostile, uncooperative, cooperative, passive	An active partner
Role of Professional	Expert responsible for care	Partner in an equal relationship
	Monitors the progress of the client toward specified goals	Engages the client in a collaborative effort
	Routine or ritualistic contact	Maintains continuous contact as needed
Orientation to Community	A source of obstacles and barriers that must be individually negotiated	A resource that can provide work, relationships and recreational opportunities
	Integration based on client's progress	Maximum integration throughout service

the outcome is a linear approach to the characteristics of the individual or the environmental factors perceived to be creating the problem. Attention focuses on defining the problem so as to specify the intervention.

The relationship of problem-solving to intervention suggests that people's inability to cope leads to a need for help from a professional with answers and resources. In the mental health system, this is exemplified by regularly scheduled, in-office counseling sessions to monitor client compliance with treatment plans and medication regimes that address symptoms of a problem. The labeling of problems distinguishes people with problems from those without them and provides roles for social workers. The barriers created by labels perpetuate dependency and a professional emphasis on failings that often result in individualistic rather than ecological accounts of human predicaments.

Second, the analysis suggests that the assumptions underlying the strengths perspective are more compatible with the philosophical base of social work than those of the problem orientation. The social work profession has consistently articulated the importance of "engaging positive forces in the person and the environment" (Germain & Gitterman, 1980, p. 19). However, supporting the dignity and worth of people along with the belief in individual and collective strength cannot be accomplished in the process of assessing liabilities. The strengths perspective transcends these limitations and attempts to lessen the gap between the profession's espoused values and actual practices.

To illustrate this point, consider the social work concepts of person-in-environment, self-determination, and maximizing potentials. Each of these, with their concern for conditions and processes that support growth, is enhanced by the strengths perspective. The enhancement of social work principals, in turn, minimizes the gap between the profession's values and actual practice methods.

How can the philosophical framework of the strengths perspective be applied to a model for social work practice? The initial step is to understand the crucial concepts of the strengths perspective, including empowerment, suspension of disbelief, dialogue and collaboration, membership, synergy, and regeneration. As illustrated in Figure 1.1, a linchpin in the new practice model is the concept of empowerment. There are two primary elements of empowerment, the psychological state and the behavioral state. The psychological state of empowerment is an increased sense of power or control over one's life situations.

Empowerment as a behavioral state uses personal power to affect change in others and to change social institutions (Gutierrez, 1990). Consequently, the process of empowerment transpires on the individual, interpersonal, and institutional levels and involves obtaining and using.

In social work vernacular, empowerment usually means to return a voice to silenced or disenfranchised people. The strengths perspective reenergizes the concept of empowerment by striving to discover the power within people and supporting the self-determined actions through the increase of self-efficacy or "the belief in one's ability to regulate life events," the development of group consciousness, the reduction of self-blame, and the assumption of personal responsibility for change (Gutierrez, 1990, p. 150). Consequently, "empowering a client is dependent upon the social worker's willingness to relinquish his or her power to create the client's context of meaning" (Weick, 1983, p. 470).

The first step in the process of empowerment is the practitioner's suspension of disbelief, defined as encouraging "the emergence of the client's truth and interpretive slant" of given situations (Saleebey, 1992, p. 13). Historically, professionals have sometimes doubted the veracity of clients, assuming that the client's views came from faulty perceptions. This suspension of belief originates from scientific investigation that

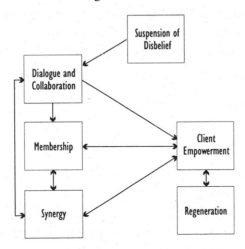

FIGURE I.I *Concepts of the strengths perspective: Foundations for a strengths model of practice*

values objective and dispassionate observations. The strengths perspective challenges reliance solely on professional expertise by emphasizing the role of clients in defining and directing change in their realities. Thus, suspension of disbelief enhances the personal power of clients by reconceptualizing the role of the professional and recognizing that people know what is best for them.

Moving toward suspension of disbelief positively influences the strengths perspective's concept of dialogue and collaboration between clients and social workers. Rappaport (1990) concluded that collaboration from a strengths perspective occurs when the social worker becomes the client's agent, consultant, or stakeholder in whatever projects or goals that are undertaken. In a collaborative relationship, the social worker and the client seek to discover the individual and communal resources that will best facilitate the achievement of the client's wants or goals (Weick, Rapp, Sullivan, & Kisthardt, 1989).

Continuous dialogue is the tool used by both parties to facilitate the collaborative process. A critical factor is client-centeredness or "starting where the client is" (Rogers, 1942). The principles of client-centeredness embrace the values of the social work profession by assuring the "client's values, needs, and individuality will take precedent and that his or her rights will prevail" (Goldstein, 1983, p. 268). Within this context, the social worker is not a passive participant. Rather, as the client's story unfolds, the social worker attends more to the client's immediate situation, the events that are currently happening and what is forecast for the future, rather than an analysis of personal history. Thus, both social workers and clients become teachers and learners in discovering what might constitute a more autonomous and rewarding way of life (Goldstein, 1983).

From collaboration and dialogue grows a sense of membership. People without membership are extremely vulnerable due to their lack of supportive networks within communities of interest and care (Saleebey, 1992). The strengths perspective recognizes the client–social worker relationship as primary and essential. From this relationship, the client begins to experience success in collaborative efforts and gains confidence to renew or initiate links to community resources.

The next step in the process of empowerment involves synergy constituted by the coming together of person and community. The notion of synergy assumes that when phenomena, including people, engage in interrelationships, "they create new and often unexpected patterns and resources that typically exceed the complexity of their individual constituents" (Saleebey, 1992, p. 11). The strengths perspective concludes that synergy involves the creation of community or group accomplishments greater than those of individuals' accomplishments. Synergy between the client and worker occurs when there is a relationship based on reciprocity, a common purpose, and joint recognition of the community as a resource.

Regeneration is the final concept of the strengths perspective. Similarly to suspension of disbelief, and collaboration and dialogue, regeneration assumes the capacity for change is inherent in people and can be self-motivated. This perspective is a radical departure from problem and pathological orientations. Instead of looking for external forces, such as a professional, to heal or solve a dilemma, attention turns to the innate abilities of clients (Weick, 1983).

Change is critical to the strengths perspective. For clients the change involves assuming an active role in determining the course of the helping encounter, recognizing aspirations as attainable, and learning to identify and use available resources. Similarly, the strengths perspective redirects the social workers' attention from problems, weaknesses or deficits to individual strengths, aspirations and interests of clients. Additional change results when the social worker views the client as a primary partner as opposed to an adversary.

Summary

A common belief is that since older individuals do not use mental health services, they do not have mental health issues (Kermis, 1986). This assumption is incorrect. For example, depression is considered the most common mental challenge of later life, yet it is not often recognized in older people. Some of the obvious signs of depression are general disinterest in activities of life, loss of appetite, and sleep disturbances

(Butler, Lewis, & Trey, 1991). Unfortunately, for older individuals depression is often confused with the mourning process and the sense of loss associated with senescence.

Related to depression is suicide. The incidence of suicide is increasing in later life, with older persons having a suicide rate three times that of the general population. Particularly at risk for suicide are older men whose retirements are often followed by social isolation and financial decline. Some older individuals are also at risk in relation to alcoholism. Currently there is a dearth of information concerning alcoholism and older people although research indicates that 10 to 15% of the aging population are faced with alcohol-related issues.

To address the mental issues of older adults, this book introduces a model for social work practice. This model is built on the conceptual components of the strengths perspective: suspension of disbelief, dialogue and collaboration, membership, synergy, and regeneration, which lead to empowerment. The strengths perspective is not compatible with social work's historic commitments, values, and principles. However, a focus on strengths urges social workers to reconsider their views of change, the client–social worker role, and the importance of relationship in the change process.

REFERENCES

Beers, C. W. (1923). *A mind that found itself.* New York: Doubleday.

Butler, R., Lewis, M., & Trey, S. (1991). *Aging & mental health: Positive psychosocial and biomedical approaches* (4th ed.). New York: Merrill Press.

DiNitto, D. (1991). *Social welfare politics and public policy.* New Jersey: Prentice Hall.

Edinberg, M. (1985). *Mental health practice with the elderly.* New Jersey: Prentice-Hall.

Foucault, M. (1965). *Madness and civilization: A history of insanity in the age of reason.* New York: Pantheon.

Germain, C., & Gitterman, A. (1980). *The life model of social work practice.* New York: Columbia University Press.

Goldman, H. H. , Adams, H. H., & Taube, C. A. (1983). Deinstitutionalization: The data demythologized. *Hospital and Community Psychiatry, 34*(2), 129–134.

Goldstein, H. (1983). Starting where the client is. *Social Casework: The Journal of Contemporary Social Work,*. May, 267 275.

Grob, G. (1966). *The state and the mentally ill: A history of Worcester State Hospital in Massachusetts, 1830–1920.* Chapel Hill: University of North Carolina Press.

Grob, G. (Ed.). (1980). *Mental hygiene in the twentieth century.* New York: Arno Press.

Gutierrez, L. M. (1990). Working with women of color: An empowerment perspective. *Social Work, 35*(2), 149–153.

Hepworth, D., & Larsen, J. A. (1990). *Direct social work practice: Theory and skills* (3rd ed.). Chicago: Dorsey.

Kermis, M. D. (1986). *Mental health in late life: The adaptive process.* Boston: Jones & Bartlett.

Kramer, M., Taube, C. A., & Redick, R.W. (1973). Patterns of use of psychiatric facilities by the aged: Past, present, and future. In C. Eisdorfer & M. F. Lawton (Eds.), *Psychology of adult development and aging,* 428–509. Washington, DC: American Psychological Association.

Mechanic, D. (1989). *Mental health and social policy* (3rd ed.). New Jersey: Prentice-Hall.

Perlman, H. H. (1957). *Social casework: A problem-solving process.* Chicago: University of Chicago Press.

Rapp, C. A. (1992). The strengths perspective of case management with persons suffering from severe mental illness. In D. Saleebey (Ed.), *The strengths perspective in social work practice,* 45–58. New York: Longman.

Rapp, C. A., & Chamberlain, R. (1985). Case management for the chronically mentally ill. *Social Work, 30*(5), 417–422.

Rappaport, J. (1990). Research methods and the empowerment agenda. In P. Tolan, C. Keys, F. Chertak, and L. Jason (Eds.), *Researching community psychology,* 127–142. Washington, DC: American Psychological Association.

Reynolds, B. (1951). *Social work and social living: Explorations in philosophy and practice.* Silver Spring, MD: National Association of Social Workers.

Robinson, V. P. (1930). *A changing psychology in social casework.* Chapel Hill: University of North Carolina.

Rogers, C. R. (1942). *Counseling and psychotherapy.* Boston: Houghton Mifflin.

Saleebey, D. (Ed.). (1992). *The strengths perspective in social work practice.* New York: Longman.

Shulman, L. (1979). *The skills of helping individuals and groups.* Chicago, IL: F. E. Peacock.

Smalley, R. E. (1967). *Theory for social work practice.* New York: Columbia University Press.

Speer, D. C., Williams, J., West, H., & Dupree, L. (1991). Older adult users of outpatient mental health services. *Community Mental Health Journal*, 27(1), 69–75.

Sue, S. (1977). Psychological theory and implications for Asian Americans. *Personnel and Guidance Journal*, 55 381–389.

Turner, F. J. (1986). *Social work treatment: Interlocking theoretical approaches.* New York: Macmillan Co.

Weick, A. (1983). Issues in overturning a medical model of social work. *Social Work, 28,* 467–471.

Weick, A., Rapp, C., Sullivan, P W., & Kishardt, W. (1989). A strengths perspective for social work practice. *Social Work, 34,* 350–354.

Zastrow, C. (1993). *Introduction to social work and social welfare.* Pacific Grove, CA: Brooks/Cole Publishing.

CHAPTER TWO

A Strengths Model of Social Work Practice

THIS CHAPTER EXAMINES THE FOUNDATION of knowledge and value base for a strengths model of social work practice. Its purpose is to define a theoretical strengths model and describe social work practice from a strengths perspective.

Included in the chapter are major features that make the strengths model unique. For example, the model is oriented toward assessing and building on strengths of individuals, groups, and communities. This does not mean that problem identification is overlooked but rather that strengths guide the selection and course of intervention. Consequently, the method of assessing and building on strengths is flexible in its application and is intended for use with other approaches including clinical interventions.

Another feature of the strengths model is its unifying effect on micro, mezzo, and macro systems (Bronfenbrenner, 1979; Magnusson & Allen, 1983). Instead of considering these levels of practice as discrete entities, the strengths model recognizes that "each level is embedded in the higher levels, and the functioning of each level is largely determined by its interaction with the higher level" (Compton & Galaway, 1994, p. 97). The result is an interconnecting process that links strengths with a sense of empowerment. This is especially critical for older individuals with mental challenges, who experience both the discrimination associated with ageism and the stigma of a mental health label.

The Foundation of Knowledge

Social work's foundation of knowledge is dynamic and reflects an understanding of biology, social sciences, and learning theories. Knowledge about people and the social environment is a cornerstone of social work practice (Germain, 1973). With a person-in-environment focus, the strengths model uses ecological theory to conceptualize practice (Council of Social Work Education, 1983). Table 2.1 defines the terms and principles of this theory in the context of a strengths perspective.

There are several reasons for selecting the ecological theory as a basis of knowledge for the strengths model. As indicated by Table 2.1, the social environment involves the circumstances, conditions, and interpersonal interactions that allow people to survive and thrive in often hostile environments. Included in the concept of social environments are the types of homes people live in, their financial resources, and the social rules and governmental laws that govern behavior and societal expectations.

Another reason the strengths model of practice uses the ecological theory is its focus on living, dynamic interaction and the active participation of people in their environment. Active participation reflects the individuality of people and presents opportunities for personal growth, mutual support, and an array of relationships.

The strengths model recognizes that reciprocity occurs in the form of interdependence. For example, an older individual volunteers to tutor in a neighborhood school. The older person with depression benefits from the one-on-one relationship with a child and maintains community involvement through the school system. The outcomes are reciprocal. Specifically, the signs of depression decrease while the child's learning opportunities increase. A significant outcome is the communication and interaction that follow. For older people, reciprocity is a critical link to remaining engaged in the activities of life.

A final reason the ecological theory is used with the strengths model involves the value of transactions as a forum to build on the strengths of informal and formal support systems. For older adults with persistent mental disorders, transactions indicate specific services

TABLE 2.1 *Applying the Strengths Model to Ecological Concepts*

TERM	ECOLOGICAL CONCEPT	STRENGTHS MODEL
Social Environment	Conditions, circumstances, and interactions of people	Involves the community and interpersonal relationships as resources that are supportive of growth and development
Person-in-Environment	People's dynamic interactions with systems	Provides a sense of continuous membership and connectedness
Transactions	Positive and negative communications between others in their environment	Fosters dialogue and collaboration to strengthen formal and informal support systems
Energy	The natural power generated from interaction between people and their environments	Results in reciprocity that creates new patterns and resources
Interface	Specific point where an individual interacts with the environment	Recognizes that intervention begins in individualized realities
Coping	Adaptation in response to a problematic situation	Highlights the innate ability of people to change and be self-motivated
Interdependence	Mutual reliance of people to one another and their environment	Occurs in relationships based on reciprocity, a common purpose, and recognition of the community as a resource

and/or environments that nurture support for the person in times of crisis as well as in times of strength. Consequently, exploring and defining transactions help to reveal how a person has survived the often harsh realities of life.

Intrinsic to the ecological theory of the strengths model of practice is a dual commitment to deliver services in collaboration with clients and to confront dysfunctional service and support systems that thwart client development. The concepts of ecological theory employed in the strengths model result in client-driven rather than provider-driven roles, routines, and rules. Consequently, "the dignity of a person transcends the role of the client in relation to any service provider" (Rose, 1992, p. 273). Further, the strengths model uses diagnosis as a descriptive rather than prescription tool.

Empowerment is an underlying element of the strengths model. The model's emphasis on collaboration, acknowledging individual realities, and recognizing unique strengths gives voice to people who have been silenced by systems of care. With a voice heard by service providers, clients discover their power to influence and direct the course of their lives (Rappaport, 1981). Empowerment underpins the strengths model's view of people as active participants in service delivery, not objects to be managed, diagnostic categories, or passive consumers of service menus.

The Value Base

Along with a specific knowledge base, the strengths model of social work practice involves values or judgments about what is important, valuable, and desirable. These values focus on "a commitment to human welfare, social justice, and individual dignity" (Reamer, 1987, p. 801). Table 2.2 applies the core values of social work to a strengths model of practice.

Beginning with respect for the dignity and uniqueness of individuals, the values of the strengths model view people holistically in the context of their social environments. Therefore, the arena for providing services extends beyond the office to the community, with practice occurring where clients live and work. For older adults with mental disorders this is significant for several reasons. First, it suggests the environment is a resource for growth and development despite conditions presented by age and mental challenges. Second, shifting the site of services from an agency location to the social environment of older people minimizes the possibility of isolation and fosters the process of

TABLE 2.2   *Applying the Values of Social Work to the Strengths Model*

VALUE	STRENGTHS MODEL
Dignity and Uniqueness of Individual	Demonstrates interest and respect for client's attributes, abilities, desires, accounts, and resources
Self-determination	Defines the social worker as collaborator or consultant who supports clients as experts of their situations
Confidentiality	Acknowledges the authenticity of client's stories, beliefs, and needs by maintaining the private nature of information
Advocacy	Supports people and their capabilities as change agents in social environments
Accountability	Assesses, with clients, how practice, services, and systems directly relate to clients' lives
Institutional Approach	Attaches no stigma to receiving funds and services. Focuses on the environmental factors associated with life conditions

empowerment, including membership, active decision making, and ongoing access to services.

Directly linked to the value of respect for the dignity and uniqueness of individuals is self-determination. In the strengths model, the perceived power of the practitioner is leveled by putting the client's needs ahead of the professional's desire for progress or an agency's menu of services. Working in a partnership connotes a new definition of the role of clients and social workers in the helping process. Qualities such as reduction of social distance, authenticity, and mutuality are emphasized when clients are asked what they need or want and what works for them (Germain & Gitterman, 1980; Rose, 1992). Oftentimes life experiences and events are instruments of change rather than techniques employed by the practitioner on the client.

An individual's right to privacy is integral to American culture, and confidentiality is an important principle of ethics critical to the strengths model. According to Lowenberg and Dolgroff (1988) confidentiality means that a social worker "will not reveal to anyone information that he/she has received on a confidential basis" (p. 74). This does not mean that social workers do not have the duty to warn and the duty to report a large number of situations involving potential danger to self or others (Compton & Galaway, 1994). Rather, the strengths model supports the obligation of social workers to clearly discuss with the client what information must be shared with whom and why. This approach to confidentially assumes clients take responsibility for their moral behaviors, including oral statements.

The strengths model views confidentiality as a commitment social workers have toward clients that reflects genuineness and consideration. In this context, confidentiality is a resource that supports open communication between clients and their informal and formal support systems.

Relationship is a condition of social work (Compton & Galaway, 1994). For older people with mental illness, the social worker is often the human link to a system of services. The relationship of the social worker and the client, built on confidentiality and self-determination, personalizes the service delivery and represents a fundamental resource of the strengths model.

An important method or technique of the strengths model is individual and systems advocacy. Individual advocacy refers to activities on behalf of an individual that often address the accessibility, availability, and adequacy of services. In comparison, systems advocacy involves addressing issues that affect groups of clients or potential clients. In either form, advocacy involves resistance and subsequent efforts to change the status quo (Kirst-Ashman & Hull, 1993). The strengths model of practice embraces advocacy as a way to mediate the inevitable conflict between people and institutions and to expand network systems. Further, advocacy activities present opportunities for clients to express and help themselves through involvement in their environment.

Implied in the value of advocacy is social action with a dual focus on persons and the environment. Successful social action efforts often link clients to desired services while influencing systems to expand resources networks. For example, an older adult with a history of institutionalization desires suitable community housing; however, subsidized housing for older people discriminates against people with mental disorders. Social action activities would address the client's need for housing on the community level and work toward institutional changes in housing policy.

Considering the dynamic nature of the strengths model, accountability is a critical value to insure a collective and continuous review of the helping process (Kishardt, 1992). In a general sense, accountability is the process of evaluating the effectiveness of services to achieve desirable goals. Specific to the strengths model, accountability involves teaching clients to monitor their own roles and functions in the helping process. The result is that clients have personal recognition and reinforcement of their achievements and opportunities to make necessary modifications in their goals and strategies. This empowers clients to exert control over their lives and assertively request assistance whenever necessary.

According to Wilensky and Lebeaux (1965) there are two views of the role of social welfare. One is the residual role, which supports the provision of social services only when all individual efforts or assets have failed or are depleted. Associated with residual services is the belief that individual deficits or inadequacies are the root of social problems. A stigma is attached to service provision based on a residual orientation.

In contrast, an institutional approach to social welfare involves no stigma because services are viewed as an entitlement of all citizens. Associated with this orientation is the belief that environmental factors cause or complicate the majority of personal difficulties. The institutional view is an integral value of the strengths model. The model recognizes the positive and negative influence of the environment on individuals and highlights people's entitlement to services that elicit, understand, and develop strengths.

The Strengths Model of Practice

Historically, social work has philosophically and theoretically recognized client strengths as a building block of assessment and intervention.

Perlman's (1957) casework model included client potential as a key component, and Ripple (1964) highlighted client motivation as a strength of effective program development. In 1971, Schwartz introduced an interactional approach to social work practice that included the belief in the strengths and health of people to address difficult life situations.

Germain and Gitterman (1980) advanced method integration with the ecological perspective currently referred to as the life model approach that (a) conceptualized the ecological perspective with a simultaneous focus on people and environments and (b) described a practice model that "integrates practice principles and skills for work with individuals, families and groups within an organizational, community, and cultural context" (Germain & Gitterman, 1986, p. 619). The life model views people's problems as outcomes of stressful person-environment relationships; however, it does not make client strengths a focal point of the assessment process.

PERSONS AND ENVIRONMENTS

As indicated by Figure 2.1, elements of the life model's ecological perspective are used to conceptualize the strengths model. In particular, the strengths model begins with persons and environments where the goodness-of-fit is a critical element linked to social class and psychosocial, social, cultural, and biological adaptive processes.

According to Germain and Gitterman (1986), the environment consists of layers, including the social and physical environment and textures, represented by time and space. The strengths model adds economic forces to the concept of environment to emphasize the psychological and social dynamics embedded in economic relations. For example, mental illnesses are often triggered by stress associated with unemployment, financial insecurity, or retirement. Examining these dynamics with clients fosters "client self-determination by engaging in exploration of societal induced constraints on human growth and development as well as individual strengths" (Burghardt, 1986, p. 608).

By recognizing the impact of economic forces on individual conditions and options, the client's individual concerns are joined with

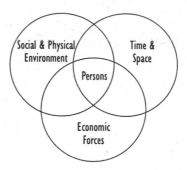

FIGURE 2.1 *Strengths model conceptualization of persons and environment*

collective ones. Consequently, micro social work intervention combines with macro practice as the client begins to place demands on the larger society for change and support. The strengths model engages social workers and clients in forms of empowerment by undermining the notion that people at various levels of income or retired from employment must settle for less than desirable benefits or conditions. Thus, from the onset, the strengths model connects individual conditions to a broader program of change.

COLLABORATIVE ASSESSMENT

In the helping professions, assessment is a process that leads to an intervention. Generally, a practitioner interviews a client to ascertain the details of problematic situations, places the information in the context of a theoretical approach, and plans strategies to alleviate the problem or its symptoms. Consequently, the majority of the helping relationship is based on the practitioner "doing for" or serving the client. Often the result is client passivity and paternalistic practice.

In contrast, the strengths model of practice, as illustrated in Figure 2.2, views assessment as an opportunity to engage the client in active programming by collaboratively defining why the client is seeking assistance and what form the assistance will take. Assessment in the strengths model involves two components, process and product (Cowger, 1992). These components are considered dynamic, requiring ongoing collaborative review and revision of client strengths and supports along with conditions.

The idea that assessment is a collaborative venture supports the social work value of self-determination and attends to the relationship between the practitioner and client. Collaborative assessment occurs when (a) engagement is viewed as a distinct activity that constitutes the initial step in developing a relationship, (b) the relationship of the practitioner and client is recognized as essential to the helping process, (c) dialogue focuses on the accomplishments and potential of the client; (d) directives and desires of clients are addressed and not judged; and (e) mutual trust is discussed, acted upon and felt by the client and practitioner.

As depicted in Figure 2.2, collaborative assessment presents a holistic portrait of clients by defining individual strengths and supports in the context of life conditions. Understanding the interrelated aspects of strengths and life conditions is vital to rediscovering personal and environmental potential, a feature of the strengths model.

STRENGTHS

Recognizing and defining client strengths is central to collaborative assessment. For people accustomed to labels and a problem focus, articulating strengths requires reeducation and reinforcement. Ideas to enhance this process include the following:

1. Considering engagement as a distinct function of the client-practitioner relationship. The notion of a formal interview is replaced by more casual, informal discussions of the client's life experiences, wants, and needs. This does not mean interview skills are not used, rather such skills are employed to foster a non-threatening atmosphere for communication.

2. Posing the question "What skills has the client used to progress and survive in life?" Behaviors often considered negative, such as manipulation and resistance, should be viewed from a positive perspective. In this light, manipulation translates into creativity or resourcefulness, and resistance correlates with independence.

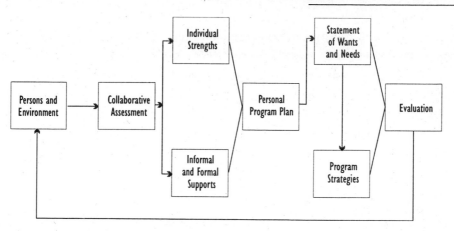

FIGURE 2.2 *Strengths model of social work practice*

3. Identifying the optimal capacity of each client to share in the responsibility of formulating life goals and designing and implementing appropriate strategies (Rose, 1992).

4. Restricting the use of diagnostic categories to descriptive information rather than prescriptive behavior and direction.

5. Moving from behind the desk and out of the agency office to meet the client in convenient community locations. Office contact should be the exception, not the rule.

Emphasizing the strengths of clients is valuable for several reasons. First, strengths are useful building blocks on which to develop interventions that anticipate positive outcomes. Reinforcing strengths in this way demonstrates respect for clients and establishes a line of communication between the client and practitioner for positive feedback.

Focusing on strengths releases clients from the stereotypes associated with labels, categories, and classifications. Although descriptors are often tied to financial reimbursement and service eligibility, their contribution to individualized assessment and program planning seldom adds clarity to the concerns, wants, and possibilities of clients. Finally, establishing strengths as the centerpiece of the assessment process is fundamental to the core of social work practice. It levels the power of the practitioner over clients and opens opportunities for partnership in the process (Cowger, 1992).

Jones and Biesecker (1980) suggest eight specific areas of consideration in defining client strengths: (a) special interests; (b) family and friends; (c) religion and values; (d) occupation and education; (e) reaction to professional services; (f) emotional and mental health; (g) physical condition; and (h) support. Over the course of conversation, the idea is to collaboratively explore and capitalize upon these potential areas of strengths in program strategies and goals.

INFORMAL AND FORMAL SUPPORT SYSTEMS

The strengths model considers people's informal and formal supports systems as resources. Informal supports, defined as family members, friends, and group affiliations offering regular or occasional emotional and/or material support, involve the client's expectation toward others. Two goals of collaborative assessment are to determine (a) the current strengths and capabilities of the informal support system and (b) the kinds of assistance the systems require to enhance or maintain their involvement with the client. This is accomplished primarily through discussions on the following:

- Who comprises the client's family members and friends and how capable are they to meet the client's needs and wants?
- In what ways does the informal system interact with other informal systems and with the client?
- In what ways does the informal system support the client?
- What are the client's community affiliations?
- What are the community's expectations for the client?

Underlying these questions are assumptions concerning the role of informal support systems and the community. The strengths model considers a person's well-being to be largely determined by the resources of the community and informal supports. Further, the model advocates that clients have a right to the resources they need for quality of life (Davidson & Rapp, 1976; Rappaport, 1977; Rapp, 1992). For this reason, informal systems and communities are recognized as untapped resources with abundant potentials for clients.

It is the practitioner's responsibility to document gaps in community and informal systems as a method to insure and advocate for necessary shifts in resource allocation. This responsibility supports the work of McKnight (1994), who suggested that "community guides" be designated to "help people to be introduced to and attached to individuals and groups within communities" (p. 430). Effective guides incorporate some of the following elements in their work:

- A focus on the gifts and capacities of excluded people
- Relationships based on trust rather than the authority of systems
- A belief that the community is hospitable to strangers
- Connections to associational life (McKnight, 1992, p. 57)

Formal systems refer to human service agencies, employment settings, and other organizations a client might contact on a regular basis. Collaborative assessment of formal systems focuses on three aspects: availability, acceptability, and accessibility (Rose, 1992; Kirst-Ashman & Hull, 1993). Availability pertains to services that match a person's needs or wants. To determine availability, a client's needs or wants must be made known and resources must be on hand to meet the stated need.

Acceptability of services is often applied to a continuum ranging from high to low. Sometimes clients refuse particular services because of past experiences or an attached stigma. At other times, services are considered highly acceptable because of the personality, techniques, and/or interpersonal skills of the service provider. Thus, acceptability of services depends on availability of services matched with the perceptions and needs of the client.

Accessibility to services involves how the environment supports a person's need for resources that are necessary for or complement services such as transportation, physical structures, or equipment. Without these necessary supports, even the most available acceptability services elude a client.

Personal Program Plan

The information gathered though collaborative assessment is compiled in the strengths model's personal program plan, a tool of the helping process. The purpose of the plan is to document a clear statement of client wants along with strategies that transform wants into realities. The planning and implementation of the personal program plan are shared activities between the client and the practitioner.

Intrinsic to the personal program plan is the belief that people have "inherent capacity to learn, grow and change" (Kisthardt, 1992). In a similar fashion, the personal program plan is dynamic and changes to reflect the attention of the practitioner because it is concrete proof of the collaborative relationship.

Two components are represented in the personal program plan: the statement of wants and program strategies. The actual formation of these components might vary from individual to individual and within the context of particular life conditions. However, the philosophy of empowerment and maximizing client self-direction are consistent features of the plan.

Statement of Wants

The statement of wants is derived by reframing clients' problems into terms of what they would like to see happen in their lives. According to Rapp (1992), three objectives are accomplished by this strategy: (a) the personal program plan addresses areas the client is motivated to work on, (b) short-term goals are defined in measurable terms, and (c) the program plan serves as a tool to monitor the behavior of the client and the practitioner in regard to completing specific tasks.

When stating wants, it is helpful to detail desirable outcomes. As clients begin to achieve outcomes, they are likely to experience a sense of accomplishment, increased motivation, and renewed confidence in their ability to control aspects of life. In many ways, the same sense of accomplishment is experienced by practitioners as they witness the success of the helping relationship.

Strategies

With the statement of wants completed, attention turns to the approaches or strategies to achieve desired outcomes. The selected strategies of the personal program serve as the routes to achieve personalized wants. Although strategies are often modified by the client and practitioner, they provide a constant focus on what is important and provide an avenue to use personal strengths to experience successes in life.

The process of selecting strategies is important to the helping relationship. Associated with the selection are a series of questions: Is this strategy one the client can implement alone? How can elements of the client's support systems assist in the strategy? How much responsibility should the practitioner assume in relation to the strategy? What is the implementation time frame for the strategy? (Kisthardt & Rapp, 1992). To answer these questions, the practitioner and client must evaluate individual strengths and systems of support in the context of the statement of wants.

Evaluation

Evaluation is emphasized throughout the strengths model as a system of accountability between practitioner and the client. Accountability refers to the mutual obligation between the two to accomplish what they have agreed upon according to negotiated time lines. The purpose of evaluation is to monitor the personal program plan and assure that designated activities are accomplishing intended goals in an effective manner.

In terms of monitoring, the evaluation process assesses the adequacy of efforts directed toward achieving client-directed goals. The information gathered from this form of evaluation focuses on the helping relationship as a means of accomplishing established goals and indicates the success of the collaboration between the practitioner and client.

The process of evaluation is directly linked to the specifications provided in strategy design. For example, if a client was to obtain housing within six months, the program plan should reflect the incremental steps to achieve this desire along with a time frame. Time frames, used as benchmarks of progress, keep evaluation process relevant to the interactions of the helping relationships.

Summary

This chapter examines the foundation of knowledge and value base of the strengths model of practice. Key concepts such as the ecological theory, the person-in-environment, self-determination, and advocacy are discussed. These concepts provide a backdrop for the presentation of the strengths model of practice.

The strengths model of practice is described as nonlinear, reflecting the chaos and challenges of life. The major components of the model—person-in-environment, collaborative assessment, the personal program plan, and evaluation—are defined. Several elements associated with the major components are identified, including strengths, informal and formal systems of support, the statement of wants, and strategies.

Finally, the chapter highlights the strengths model's hallmark as its focus on strengths in the assessment phase. The model's approach to change integrates the wants of individuals to societal shifts in the allocation of resources. Thus, the strengths model includes the notion that clients and practitioners are change agents working in collaboration.

References

Bronfenbrenner, V. (1979). *The ecology of human development*. Cambridge, MA: Harvard University Press.

Burghardt, S. (1986). Marxist theory and social work. In F. Turner (Ed.), *Social work treatment: Interlocking theories* (pp. 590–617). New York: The Free Press.

Compton, B. A., & Galaway, B. (1994). *Social work processes*. Pacific Grove, CA: Brooks/Cole Publishing.

Council of Social Work Education. (1983). *Curriculum policy for masters degree and baccalaureate degree programs in social work education*. New York: Author.

Cowger, C. D. (1992). Assessment of clients. In D. Saleebey (Ed.), *The strengths perspective in social work practice* (pp. 139–147). New York, NY: Longman.

Davidson W. & Rapp, C. (1976). Child advocacy in the justice system. *Social Work, 21* (3), 225–232.

Germain, C. B. (1973). An ecological approach to people-environment transactions. *Social Casework, 62*(6), 323–331.

Germain, C. B., & Gitterman, A. (1980). *The life model of social work practice*. New York: Columbia University Press.

Germain, C. B., & Gitterman, A. (1986). The life model approach to social work revisited. In F. Turner (Ed.), *Social work treatment: Interlocking theories* (pp. 618–644). New York: The Free Press.

Jones, M., & Biesecker, J. (1980). Goal planning in child and youth services. DDHS Publication No. (OHDS) 81-30295. Washington, DC: US Government Printing Office. In B. R. Compton & B. Galaway (Eds.), 1994. *Social work processes* (pp. 223–224). Pacific Grove, CA: Brooks/Cole Publishing.

Kirst-Ashman, K. K. & Hull, G H. (1993). *Understanding generalist practice*. Chicago: Nelson-Hall.

Kisthardt, W. E. & Rapp, C. A. (1989). Bridging the gap between principles and practice: Implementing a strengths perspective in case management. In D. Saleebey (Ed.), 1992. *The strengths perspective in social work practice*. White Plains, NY: Longman Publishing, p. 59.

Kisthardt, W. E. (1992). A strengths model of case management: The principals and functions of a helping partnership with persons with persistent mental illness. In D. Saleebey (Ed.), *The strengths perspective in social work practice* (pp. 59–83). New York: Longman.

Lowenberg, F. & Dolgroff, R. (1988). *Ethical decisions for social work practice*. Itasca, Illinois: F. E. Peacock.

Magnusson, D. & Allen, V. L. (1983). *Human development: An interactional perspective*. New York: Academic Press.

McKnight, J. (1992). Redefining community. *Social Policy, 23*, pp. 56–62.

McKnight, J. (1994). Do no harm: Policy options that meet human needs. In B. R. Compton & B. Galaway (Eds.). *Social work processes*. Pacific Grove, California: Brooks/Cole, pp. 565–571.

Perlman, H. H. (1957). *Social casework: A problem-solving process*. Chicago: University of Chicago Press.

Rapp, C. A. (1992). The strengths perspective of case management with persons suffering from severe mental illness. In D. Saleebey (Ed.), *The strengths perspective in social work practice*. New York: Longman.

Rappaport, J. (1977). *Community psychology: Values, research, and action*. New York: Holt, Rinehart and Winston.

Rappaport, J. (1981). In praise of paradox: A social policy of empowerment over protection. *American Journal of Community Psychology, 9*, 1–25.

Reamer, F. G. (1987). Values and ethics. In A. Minihan (Ed.), *Encyclopedia of Social Work, Vol. 2*, (18 ed., pp. 801–809). Silver Spring, MD: National Association of Social Workers.

Ripple, L. (1964). *Motivation, capacity and opportunity*. Chicago: University of Chicago Press.

Rose, S. M. (1992). Case management: An advocacy/empowerment design. In S. M. Rose (Ed.), *Case management and social work practice* (pp. 271–297). New York: Longman.

Schwartz, W. (1971). On the use of groups in social work practice. In W. Schwartz and S. Zalba (Eds.), *The practice of group work.* New York: Columbia University Press, pp. 3–24.

Wilensky, H. L. & Lebeaux, C. N. (1965). *Industrial society and social welfare: The impact of industrialization on the supply and organization of social welfare services in the United States.* New York : The Free Press.

~⁓〇⌒~

Conducting a Strengths Assessment and Completing a Personal Program Plan

A SSESSMENT IS A HALLMARK of social work practice. This chapter discusses the assessment process and the personal program plan in the context of the strengths model. Its purpose is to clarify how engagement, continuous collaboration, advocacy, and supportive disengagement generate a holistic profile of an individual from a strengths perspective.

The chapter illustrates how recognizing and building on strengths is an integral part of the assessment and program planning that makes the strengths model a unique practice method. Unlike Perlman's (1957) casework model, Schwartz and Zalba's (1971) interactional approach, Pincus and Minahan's (1973) problem-solving method, and the life model of Germain and Gitterman (1980), the strengths model considers strength assessment as a preeminent component of the helping process. Gathering information on potential support people, leisure activities, individual achievements, and survival skills sends a signal to people early in the helping process that growth is possible and positive outcomes are expected.

Initiating a strengths assessment requires social workers to actively engage in relationships that position the clients as experts in their life situations. Consequently, instead of searching through files and charts for data, social workers use the gathering of information as a vehicle to foster and reinforce the concept of collaboration. This is especially critical for older people whose comments and concerns are sometimes discounted because of stereotypes associated with aging. As a result of the single emphasis on strengths and resources rather than symptomatology and problems, the pressing question is not what kind of life one has but rather what kind of life one wants.

The Strengths Assessment

The assessment process gathers relevant, broad-based information. Data such as sociodemographic data and other essential information help the client and the social worker to understand the client's current status and overall environment. Equally as important is the information obtained through guided but informal discussions with the client. To capture this information in a working document, Figure 3.1 illustrates a strengths assessment form adapted from the state of Ohio's *Case Management Training Handbook* (Hyde, 1992).

The assessment holistically profiles an individual by gathering information in six life domains, including living arrangements, social supports, relationships, personal care, education, leisure and recreational activities, health, and financial resources. Within this context four dimensions are considered: current individual status, personal goals, internal and external resources, and priority of needs and wants. Following the dimensions through life domains lends a direction and flow to the assessment process and provides opportunities for collaboration with the client.

The social worker uses the strengths assessment as a template for engaging in dialogue and assisting the client to tell the story (Cowger, 1992). In total, the strengths assessment is a

1. Tool to represent the growth and changing concerns of the client
2. Map for establishing the relationship between the social worker and a client
3. Reflection of the client interacting with the environment
4. Working document with a beginning, but no end

The assessment is ongoing and updated when goals are achieved, the client's status is altered, or resources are required (Hyde, 1992). As

FIGURE 3.1 *Strengths Assessment*
Personal Program Plan

Social Worker/Case Manager's Name _____

Client's Name _____

CURRENT SITUATION: WHAT'S GOING ON NOW?	PERSONAL GOALS: WHAT I'D LIKE TO HAVE/ACHIEVE	RESOURCES: INTERNAL/EXTERNAL WHAT HAVE I USED? WHAT CAN I USE?	PRIORITIZED NEEDS/WANTS: WHAT STEPS DO I TAKE?

Living Arrangements: My living situation...

Social Supports: Who's important in my life/where can I go for support?

Social Worker/Case Manager's Name

Client's Name

| CURRENT SITUATION: WHAT'S GOING ON NOW? | PERSONAL GOALS: WHAT I'D LIKE TO HAVE/ACHIEVE | RESOURCES: INTERNAL/EXTERNAL WHAT HAVE I USED? WHAT CAN I USE? | PRIORITIZED NEEDS/WANTS: WHAT STEPS DO I TAKE? |

Relationships: How do I feel about my relationships with others (interpersonal) and my relationship with myself (intrapersonal)?

Personal Care: What activities can I do to care for myself or others?

Education: What would I like to learn?

Social Worker/Case Manager's Name

Client's Name

PERSONAL GOALS: WHAT I'D LIKE TO HAVE/ACHIEVE	RESOURCES: INTERNAL/EXTERNAL WHAT HAVE I USED? WHAT CAN I USE?	PRIORITIZED NEEDS/WANTS: WHAT STEPS DO I TAKE?

CURRENT SITUATION: WHAT'S GOING ON NOW?

Leisure/Recreation: What activities do I like/how do I spend my time?

Health: How do I stay physically and mentally healthy?

Financial: What's my money situation?

Personal Strengths List

What do I like about myself? _____
What are my strengths? _____
What assets do others think I have? _____

defined in Table 3.1, a strengths assessment is different from a traditional diagnostic assessment in purpose, format and outcome.

Specifically, the concept of clinical diagnosis evolved from a medical model of practice that primarily emphasizes interventions as a product to address pathology and deficits. In contrast, a strengths assessment is both a process and product (Hepworth and Larsen, 1982). According to Cowger (1992) the assessment process is a joint venture between the client and social worker and as a product "it is being constantly being revised during the life of the helping relationship" (p. 141).

TABLE 3.1 *Comparing a Strengths Assessment to a Diagnostic Assessment*

	STRENGTHS ASSESSMENT	DIAGNOSTIC ASSESSMENT
Goal	To collaborate with a client to identify their current needs/wants in the life domain of living arrangements, social support, relationships, personal care, education, leisure/recreation, health, and finances.	To specify problem areas of deficits, identify symptoms, and identify behavior according to DSM-IV.
Focus	Highlight areas of strengths, wants, and resources available.	Modification of primary and secondary symptoms.
Intervention	Build on strengths. Place client in the position of expert and mobilize resources to growth-oriented outcomes.	Medication is presented based upon symptoms and the DSM-IV diagnosis. Psychological therapy is available.
Outcome	A dynamic plan for client from current status toward their personal goals in each life domain.	Outcomes viewed in terms of prognosis, compliance with medication, and psychiatric stabilization.
Provider	Client with social worker.	Mental health professional.

Adapted from *Case Management Training Handbook*, by P. Hyde, 1992, Ohio Department of Mental Health.

Understanding the nature and implications of both a clinical diagnosis and a strengths assessment is critical for social workers. Each assessment has its own unique purpose, format, and outcome. An area of a diagnostic assessment that must be taken into consideration during a strengths assessment is use of the Diagnostic and Statistical Manual of Mental Disorders IV (DSM-IV). In the traditional diagnostic assessment, the mental status of the client is ascertained and remains a prescriptive element of the assessment process. The DSM-IV diagnosis is important for financial reimbursement and marks the client's entrance into local, state, and federal mental health systems. However, equally as important is the strengths assessment because it facilitates a partnership and assists clients to discover, clarify, and express their needs and their potential (Cowger, 1992).

The Social Worker's Role in a Strengths Assessment

In the strengths model of social work practice, the social worker immediately engages the client by building a secure and comfortable environment for sharing personal information. This is accomplished by empowering the client with the belief that the client has the resources and capabilities to struggle, survive, and thrive in the community. Therefore, during initial meetings, completing forms and gathering psychiatric histories are not the primary focus. Rather, discussing topics of interest to the client is encouraged by *formal and informal questions* that place the client in an expert position.

For example, during their initial meeting, the social worker asks Mrs. Jeanne Devine to describe some of her "proudest moments." Mrs. Devine pauses and states, "Well, there was a time when I would spend the majority of my spring and summer days in the garden. In fact, I started my plants from seeds and took great care to water and feed them before placing them in garden spots. The neighbors often commented on the beauty of my work. I felt proud throughout the summer whenever I thought of my garden."

Mrs. Devine's comments indicate the strength of patience and nurture. The social worker gathers information on Mrs. Devine's interests and her response to positive recognition. Gardening can be a vehicle for the social worker to ask follow-up questions on Mrs. Devine's current activities or hobbies and particular relationships with neighbors.

The strengths assessment is completed by the client in concert with the social worker. As a team they identify the client's current status, strengths, and personal goals and wants according to life domains. The information gathered is updated through regularly scheduled collaborative assessments to reflect changes in the client's life and perceptions. Through nonverbal and verbal communication the social worker recognizes the client as the expert. To accomplish this the social worker

Maintains an attitude that is positive and affirmative toward the client.

Engages in active listening as the client articulates concerns and possibilities.

Conducts meetings in environments familiar to the client, such as the home, a park, or local coffee shop.

Talks candidly about the client's behavior and interpersonal activities.

Remains nonjudgmental.

Expresses a willingness to assist the client in good times and through difficulties.

Initiates action according to the client's direction.

Throughout the strengths assessment the relationship shared by the social worker and client is primary. Consequently, mutual respect, rapport and ongoing trust are anticipated outcomes of social work services.

CONDUCTING THE STRENGTHS ASSESSMENT

The strengths assessment documents the client's words in a clear and concise manner. Difficulties associated with completing a strengths assessment fall into several major areas. First, the social worker and client must avoid problem-solving discussions that do not comment on strengths and life successes. This is sometimes difficult because social work practice often focuses on problem solving as a way to legitimize intervention and to mark progress or failure with a client. Second, positive actions and movement must be the focus of the client–social work relationship. This necessitates celebrating accomplishments, no matter how small or incremental. For people with persistent mental challenges, recognizing and appreciating success is a often a new experience that must be learned and reinforced over a period of time. Finally, the client and social worker should be mindful that a strengths assessment is an ongoing process, as is its documentation. The completion of an assessment does not occur at a specific time or date but rather reflects the commitment of the client and social worker to progressive change and monitoring.

To begin a strengths assessment, the social worker introduces himself or herself to the client and provides a brief overview of the social work process. In this initial stage, the assessment might be described as a map for identifying goals and strategies. It is important for the social worker to keep pace with the client, so the process is not rushed. The assessment is viewed as a tool rather than a form so the introduction should be relaxed for all involved and an enjoyable time when the uniqueness of the client begins to surface.

Initiate the strengths assessment by asking the client to select a life domain for completion. This immediately places the client in the decision-making role. Move from one life domain to another depending on the client's conversation. For example, if the client would like to visit more often with a particular son or daughter but is unable to do so because of physical conditions, questions can begin to flow toward the life domain of health. Portions of the health domain could be completed and then the discussion could return to the client's children (Hyde, 1992). Thus, the client and social worker are encouraged to move freely through the life domains and connect comments from one domain to another.

In the case of Harry Rose, throughout his conversation with the social worker, he expresses his fear of failing health. "I've just never been right since the last operation and that worries me. My sight seems to be going and the glasses don't do the trick. I can hardly work on my stamp collection. Did you know I was a stamp collector? Actually, I inherited a terrific collection from my father-in-law and throughout the years I've added to it. Now, my father-in-law, there was a wonderful man. He's been dead for 20 or 30 years but I can still see him sitting in a chair under that tree."

Throughout the assessment process it is critical to capture the details of the client's comments. Specifically, in the case of Mr. Rose it is important to define his visual impairment in terms of what activities are difficult and to what degree he needs assistance and medical attention. Also, it is equally as essential to document what activities the client is able to complete and how often.

Complete the assessment with short, descriptive, and nonjudgmental phrases (Hyde, 1992). Whenever possible quote the client. If feasible, encourage the client to write the entire assessment or portions of it. This empowers the client in the role of expert and reinforces the idea of social worker as learner in terms of understanding the client as a whole person.

After one or more of the life domains have been completed, the social worker and client identify the primary life domain as a beginning point to discuss goal attainments. The primary life domain should be designated based on survival needs. In the case of older adults, health conditions or living arrangements are often primary life domains. Once designated, the client and social worker discuss the needs to achieve the goal listed in the selected life domain. The following case illustrates how the needs are prioritized:

Amy Brian selects Living Arrangements as her primary life domain. Currently, Mrs. Brian resides in the family's three-story house located in a rural county seat in a Midwestern state. Since the death of her spouse, Mrs. Brian cannot maintain the house, considering her medical and financial situations. Mrs. Brian lists her needs as

PRIORITY NEEDS

1. Meet with her children (two sons and a daughter)
2. Reconstruct her house to make it more appropriate to her current medical and financial situations

PRIORITY   NEEDS

3. Discuss with friends and clergy the possibility of renting a room to a boarder

4. Explore living options including moving to a senior citizen complex or residing with her daughter

The next step was for Mrs. Brian to prioritize her needs. She accomplished this independently by numbering the needs as indicated above.

Constructing a Personal Program Plan

A personal program plan is designed to address the needs specified by clients during the strengths assessment. Adapted from the state of Ohio's *Case Management Training Handbook* (Hyde, 1992), Figure 3.2 illustrates a personal program plan as a set of action steps comprising the life domains, long-term goals, short-term goals, and strategies. The name of the person responsible for a particular strategy along with the date the strategy is to be accomplished is included in the plan to establish an ongoing monitoring system from the start. The signatures of the client, social worker, and other involved individuals suggest the personal plan is a commitment or a contract between people who agree to tasks and responsibilities.

Similar to the strengths assessment, the personal plan is completed based upon the client's stated interests. Consequently, the guidelines for completing the plan are individualized to reflect the client's situation and view of reality. Table 3.2 defines the components of the personal program plan.

The personal plan is developed with the client in conjunction with the strengths assessment or during a follow-up session (Hyde, 1992). It can be completed when the client completes the dimensions of one life domain or the entire strengths assessment. In either case, the following steps are recommended:

1. Check the box to denote the selected life domain.

2. Complete the long-term goal based upon the client's personal goal in the specific life domain listed in the strengths assessment.

FIGURE 3.2   *Personal Program Plan*

Social Worker/Case Manager's Name _____   Client's Name _____

Life Domain	___ Living Arrangements	___ Social Supports	___ Relationships	___ Personal Care
	___ Education	___ Leisure/Recreational	___ Health	___ Financial

Long-term Goal

MEASURABLE SHORT-TERM TREATMENT GOALS AND INTERMEDIATE ACTION STEPS	RESPONSIBILITY FOR ACTION PLAN: PROVIDER NAME, LICENSE INITIALS; FREQUENCY; MODALITY; REFERRALS	DATE TO BE ACCOMPLISHED	DATE COMPLETED

If more than one page, signatures are required on the last page and are optional on the other pages

Client's Signature _____   Signature and title (other) _____

Date _____   Date _____

Social Worker's Signature _____   Signature and title (other) _____

Date _____   Date _____

TABLE 3.2 *Components of a Personal Program Plan*

COMPONENT	DEFINITION
Life domain	There are eight domains representing key aspects of life. Only one life domain is checked per personal program plan. A new plan is created for each different life domain and for individual needs and wants.
Long-term goal	The goal is a restatement of the personal goal on the strengths assessment.
Strategies	Action steps that restate the prioritized needs of the strengths assessment. These steps are measurable and observable.
Responsibility for strategies	The names of individuals responsible for completing the strategy.
Date to be accomplished	The projected date to accomplish the strategy.
Date accomplished	The actual date the strategy is completed.
Comments	Statements made by the client and other individuals concerning the goal.
Signatures	The personal program plan is signed by all individuals involved with the strategy.

3. Include all people in the planning process necessary to accomplish the goal such as family members, neighbors, or physicians.

4. List the first prioritized need as a short-term goal, then design corresponding strategies to achieve the short-term goal. Strategies should be broken into small steps that the client can achieve with minimal assistance. Strategies involve skills that build upon one another.

5. Specify the person responsible for each particular step in achieving a strategy.

6. List the date each step is to be completed.

7. Document pertinent comments made by the client or other people involved in the planning process.

8. Review the plan with the client.

9. Secure signatures from all individuals involved in the planning process.

10. Indicate a minimum of contact frequency between the social worker and the client.

11. Update the personal plan on a monthly basis or as needed.

12. Develop additional personal plans for life domains or needs.

13. Recognize and celebrate the successes achieved through the personal plan.

(Adapted from *Case Management Training Handbook*, by P. Hyde, 1992, Ohio Department of Mental Health.)

The Social Worker's Role in a Personal Program Plan

Throughout the development of the personal program plan, the social worker educates and reinforces the client in the decision-making process. Older adults with mental health challenges often think they have few options in life. The role of the social worker must be to confront this misconception by emphasizing the right of clients to choose strategies that direct their lives toward personal goals.

Supporting clients as they move toward goals is a function of the social worker. This involves providing enough assistance so the clients remain in the expert position but feel the presence of the social worker as a resource. Rather than focusing on the questions needed to complete the personal plan, the social worker should consider questions as tools to encourage older adults to think and talk about issues of relevance (Kivnick, 1993). More important than the answers to specific questions is the overall pattern of life stories, values, and strengths that older adults will bring to light. Documenting these stories in the form of the personal program plan facilitates life planning and validates the strengths and behavioral expressions older adults have used to survive the uneven road of life.

When a client accomplishes one step of a strategy, the social worker should celebrate the success. Although the step may be as small as combing hair or making a telephone call, there is reason to rejoice in the accomplishment.

Paul Williams talked about his recent success with Victor Howe, social worker. "Not so long ago I couldn't ride in a car for more than a few moments without feeling closed in and nervous. But, I've been working on my breathing exercises like we agreed and yesterday I traveled to town without a major problem. To celebrate, I treated myself to a cheese steak with fried onions. What's a little fat in the diet once in awhile, especially after experiencing some success?"

Celebrations may be a simple verbal statement or more elaborate, such as a special meal. Whatever the case the emphasis is on the client's positive efforts and results. Acknowledgments are essential for the morale of both the client and social worker because they highlight progress and support expectations for positive outcomes.

Summary

Instead of thinking of old age as a social problem, the strengths model of social work introduces a strengths assessment and personal program plan to maximize human resources. As the notion of older adults' resources broaden, an understanding of the dynamics of spirit begins to emerge. Enhancing the vitality of this spirit involves social workers encouraging older adults to build on past strengths so as to move toward the future.

The purpose of the strengths assessment and the personal plan is to improve the quality of life of older adults by recognizing and building on life successes. As complementary tools, the assessment and personal plan harness the resources of individuals by connecting personal strengths to individualized needs and goals. Thus, the strengths assessment and personal plan align social work practice with its system of values (Weick, Rapp, Sullivan, & Kisthardt, 1989).

A strengths assessment is necessary to the strengths model of social work practice. The assessment focuses on the client's capabilities and aspirations in all life domains. The personal plan operationalizes the client's aspiration through a series of actions steps stated in positive terms. As a team, the client and social worker collaborate to unveil resources available within the client and the client's life.

REFERENCES

American Psychiatric Association. (1994). *The diagnostic and statistical manual of mental disorders*. Washington, DC: American Psychiatric Association.

Cowger, C. D. (1992). Assessment of client strengths. In Saleebey, D. (Ed.), *The strengths perspective in social work practice* (pp. 139–147). New York: Longman.

Germain, C., & Gitterman, A. (1980). *The life model of social work practice*. New York: Columbia University Press.

Hepworth, D. & Larsen, J. (1982). *Direct social work practice*. Homewood, IL: Dorsey Press.

Hyde, P. (1992). *Case management training handbook*. Columbus, OH: Ohio Department of Mental Health.

Kivnick, H. Q. (1993, Winter/Sping). Everyday mental health: A guide to assessing strengths. *Generations*, 13–20.

Perlman, H. (1957). *Social casework: A problem-solving process*. Chicago: University of Chicago Press.

Pincus, A., & Minahan, A. (1973). *Social work practice: Model and method*. Itasca, IL: F. E. Peacock.

Schwartz, W., & Zalba, S. (1971). *The practice of group work*. New York: Columbia University Press.

Weick, A., Rapp, C., Sullivan, W. P., & Kisthardt, W. (1989). A strengths perspective for social work practice. *Social Work*, July, 350–354.

Depression in Later Life

VOLUMES HAVE BEEN WRITTEN about depression generally, as well as about age and gender specifically. This chapter discusses depression as it relates specifically to the older adult, offering only a brief overview of the topic to provide the necessary framework for application of the strengths model.

Depression and depressive behavior are the most common mental health complaints of older people. Older persons experience much less major depression than they do secondary or reactive depression. Secondary or reactive depressions arise in response to significant life events with which the individual has difficulty coping (Hooyman & Kiyak, 1991). The reason for the difficulty is that the environment is not supportive of older people in terms of helping them cope with the ongoing stressors that accompany growing old. The focus of this chapter is on secondary and reactive depressions.

The Environment, Age, and Depression

In our youth-oriented, production-minded society, the aged have become devalued. The wisdom and experience gained through years of living is of diminishing importance to the younger generations (Osgood, 1985) as they push on to fulfill their own life goals and seek their own form of wisdom. With the high technological advances of the last 20 years, this gap of relating to new technology will continue to widen and distance the young from seeing older adults as useful or intelligent: "Grandma can't work the microwave, answering machine, computer," and so forth.

Ageism, prejudice against older people, transcends social and economic changes that have been made by older people. Cultural attitudes that reflect the idea that the seniors are not contributing members of our society hold more importance than patterns of progress made by the older adult. These attitudes, out with the old and in with the new (young) reinforce ageism. The strengths perspective confronts the notion of "useless old people" and views the aging process as normal.

Loss

From a psychological perspective, old age has been described as the season of losses, including financial, emotional, psychological, physical, and social. These are seen in the loss of a spouse, children, friends, self-esteem, self-confidence, personal control, competence, hearing, sight, physical health, mobility, job, community activities, status, power, and income (Osgood, 1985).

Loss can cause or exacerbate depression and when there are several major losses in the life of older persons, their psychological equilibrium can be compromised. The loss of a loved one is a contributor to depression, which can be a major feature of the normal grief process for many (Glick, Weiss, & Parkes, 1974; Parkes, 1965). The loss of a spouse of many years brings forth sadness and loneliness, and survivors often feel that parts of themselves have died. Life becomes seemingly empty and meaningless, and to compound that difficulty, this feeling is often accompanied by the fear and anxiety that comes when the person is faced with the prospect of living alone (Osgood, 1985). For example, a man who is older and survives the loss of a spouse may then become isolated because the spouse maintained the bridges of support within the family, such as cards, calls, birthdays, and so forth, and his lack of skill or appreciation for the importance of these bridges can lessen the resources to which he has access (Miller, 1979).

Helplessness follows on the heels of depression. Older persons' newly acquired roles, based solely on the criteria of age, change and they no longer enjoy the same status in society. Typically depressed persons do not believe that they can control those elements of life that relieve suffering or bring gratification. Older adults are more susceptible to these feelings of helplessness because they experience the greatest loss of control (i.e., child-rearing, work, income, physical health, etc.) as they move into late life (Seligman, 1975).

LONELINESS

Butler, Lewis, and Sunderland (1991) gave a developmental analogy concerning the struggles in infancy and in later life of coming to terms with loneliness. The infant experiences alternate sensations of gratifying warmth and comfort of the parent and the fear of aloneness and can become totally absorbed in a task or an action that is not dependent on another person. The character of loneliness is different in old age in that seniors have mastered their survival and provided successfully for their own physical and emotional sustenance. With older persons' diminished participation within the community and society, however, there is once again the threat of aloneness. Unlike the child, an "older person does not suffer so much from a fear of being unable to relate as from the reality of having no one to relate to" (Butler, Lewis, & Sunderland, 1991, p. 94).

Weiss (1973) described loneliness as being caused not by being alone but being without some definite needed relationship. Furthermore, he made the distinction between the loneliness of emotional isolation, the absence of a close emotional attachment leading to feelings of emptiness, and social isolation that is associated with the absence of a social network leading to feelings of boredom, rejection, and marginality (Weiss, 1973).

Characteristics of Depression: Relationship to Environment

The range of depression varies from the "blues" to loss of interest or pleasure in usual activities to thoughts of death or suicide. A person can go from a mild sense of disquiet to profound emptiness, melancholy,

and despair (Butler, et al., 1991; Osgood, 1985). Epidemiologic estimates vary as to the actual rates of major depression among the older
population, but it seems to be low, approximately 2%, but milder forms
of depression are as high as 20 to 31% (Klerman, et al., 1985; Gurland,
Dean, Cross, & Golden, 1980). Discrepancies across studies regarding
the rates of depression among older adults are partially explained by
the higher incidence of atypical symptoms, for example, increased
socioeconomic problems, concurrent medical illnesses, and changing
epidemiologic and diagnostic techniques (Ruegg, Zisook, & Swerdlow,
1988).

The concept of late life or late onset depression continues to be
debated. There is controversy as to whether the initial development of
depression after the age of 60 represents a distinct biologic subtype
(Greenwald & Kramer-Ginsberg, 1988). The controversy begs the
question: Is depression a natural component of the aging process? From
the strengths perspective, depression is seen as a normal reaction to life
conditions and occurs in older and younger adults alike. The strengths
model strives to empower older people, giving them back control of
their lives, enabling them to regain an attachment to living. For example, Mrs. M. was not depressed because her daughter lived across the
country. She was depressed because she had to quit driving as a result of
mild memory loss, she was lonely since having had to place her husband
in a nursing home, and she missed her daughter. Mrs. M. wanted
contact with her daughter and that could be accomplished. The practitioner helped to empower Mrs. M. through dialogue and collaboration
and came up with ways to make the contact with her daughter happen.
The practitioner learned that Mrs. M.'s daughter used an audio re-
corder for her work, and it was arranged that she would send her
mother audio tapes once a month and write once a month. Mrs. M. and
her daughter also agreed that they would alternate calling each other on
a weekly basis. With this plan, Mrs. M. not only felt empowered, she
experienced a regeneration by having consistent contact with her
daughter.

To further clarify this point, one might note Kermis's (1986) distinction in older adults between depression as an illness rather than as a

state of being. With the common stereotypes associated with old age, it is not unexpected that old age and depression have similar characteristics. There is a tendency for old age to mimic depression, but there are some straightforward ways to differentiate normal old age from depression.

> Although older people often worry, worry that cannot be stopped tends to indicate depression. Loneliness when not socially isolated, general rather than specific past regrets, inactivity preceded by a loss of interest, and long pauses before speaking also indicate depression rather than advanced old age. (Kermis, 1984, cited in Kermis, 1986, p. 195)

Identification of depression in the older population is often influenced by what is considered age-appropriate behavior. Trouble concentrating, poor memory, and a change in problem-solving skills, all signs of depression in younger people, are more likely to be labeled behaviors of dementia in the older person. Dementia is often not only considered but assumed given the clients advanced age (Kermis, 1986).

On average, older adults report as many depressive behaviors as do younger adults; however, they are less likely to be treated for depressive conditions (George, 1993). The reasons for the depressive behaviors of older adults, however, differ. First, older adults may be more prone to mild depression than younger adults. Sadness and occasional bouts of depression typically are normal reactions to the stressors and losses that occur in late life, such as bereavement, retirement, reduced income, and declining health. This form of depression is usually episodic and of short duration. Second, higher rates of physical illness may produce symptoms of depression. Depression frequently accompanies many chronic medical illnesses in older people, with the medical difficulties entering into the differential identification. The identification of concurrent depression and medical illness can be difficult (Butler, et al., 1991) because some practitioners discount behaviors of depression due to the physical illness (George, 1993). George (1993) asserted that the diagnostic tools used by traditional practitioners exclude behaviors that are likely to be due to physical health problems. Further, she suggested that the traditional diagnostic criteria for depressive disorders are not "age fair" because many significant depressive syndromes presented by older adults do not fit the DSM-IV-R guidelines. For example, the guidelines do not account for social and environmental factors or the availability of social support—friends and relatives who are willing and able to provide assistance (George, 1993).

Social and demographic risk factors predisposing older persons to depression are much like those found for younger persons. Women, the unmarried and particularly the widowed, and those with stressful life circumstances who lack supportive social networks are believed to be at increased risk for serious depression. Furthermore, the course of depression for older persons is similar to that in younger persons (National Institutes of Health, 1992). The racial and ethnic minorities who are generally exposed to the significant risk factors mentioned above report no more depressive symptoms than do whites (George, 1993).

TRADITIONAL INTERVENTIONS

Ageism, insufficient training, unfavorable reimbursement policies, and the absence of specific expertise for identifying depression among the older population are all factors believed to stand in the way of adequate identification of and intervention in depression in the older clients (Pollner, 1991). It has been estimated that only about 20% of patients 65 and older are provided intervention by mental health specialists.

Today's older persons are more likely to have formed their coping strategies during the Great Depression, when self-reliance was particularly prized. Social security programs did not begin until 1935, so present-day older adults did not see the older persons of their time using social services, especially for mental health. Another deterrent to seeking mental health intervention was the reputation of public mental hospitals for committing atrocities, which older adults may continue to fear. Having grown up in a time when expression of feelings and emotions may have been considered inappropriate, older clients may feel uncomfortable with the idea of discussing them.

If and when intervention is sought, dementia may be considered a more age-appropriate identification by mental health specialists than depression. For instance, where a younger client's report of sleep disturbance and difficulty concentrating may be readily attributed to depression, the same disturbances in an older person may be considered normal physical responses to the decreased need for sleep and a slowing of mental capabilities that frequently occur in advanced age. Memory complaints demonstrate a stronger association with depressed mood than with performance on memory tests (Neurol, 1991).

Antidepressants have been shown to be successful as a traditional intervention. Drug therapy is not overlooked when using the strength perspective. When properly monitored, antidepressants and counseling, sometimes in combination, restore 60 to 80% of older clients with depression back to health. However, changes in body chemistry associated with aging may cause effective intervention using antidepressants to take longer in older persons than younger persons before significant improvement is seen. Counseling (psychotherapy) also has gained more recognition recently as a successful approach in working with the older client (Hunt, 1991).

Although electroconvulsive therapy (ECT) has shown some positive results in treatment of depression among older clients, relapse is frequently reported. Limited data suggest that the older a client is, the more likely there is to be post-ECT confusion following intervention (American Family Physician, 1992). Confusion for people of all ages after ECT is common, but it is generally short-term, with complete recovery.

Applying the Strengths Model to Depression

The strengths-based model is especially viable for working with depressive behaviors because it takes clients out of a diagnostic labeling mode and places them in a holistic intervention mode. Individuals are viewed as persons, not as older or younger persons, and depressive behavior is put in the perspective of the context of their present lives with consideration given to the entire life cycle they have experienced.

For example, Mrs. Smith, age 32, and Mrs. Jones, age 79 both experienced loss, shock, denial, grief, and depression upon the death (expected or unexpected) of their husbands. The differences in their experiences would no doubt come from the way the two women were supported by the environment. In the case of Mrs. Smith, whose husband died suddenly from a cerebral hemorrhage, a referral was made to a crisis intervention center by her physician. She received individual counseling and then was referred to a bereavement support group to help her manage the grieving process. Her two young children were put in a children's bereavement group at the same center, and the counselors from each group worked together to coordinate the intervention for the family. Mrs. Smith's physician also prescribed an antidepression drug shortly after the referral to the crisis center. The assumption was that Mrs. Smith was young, had a long life ahead of her, and needed assistance in her grieving process.

In the case of Mrs. Jones, whose husband's death was expected, the type of intervention was quite different. Mrs. Jones's husband had experienced a serious illness 6 months prior to his death, was hospitalized, and subsequently placed in a nursing home. Before her husband's death and after a near fire incident in the kitchen, Mrs. Jones was moved into the home of her son and his family. Mr. Jones died 2 months later. Her son and his family were appropriately supportive. However, there was no outside intervention sought for Mrs. Jones to deal with her grief over her husband's loss, presumably because, at her age, her husband's death was just part of the aging process and she would gradually get over it. Mrs. Jones's physician also prescribed antidepression medication for her.

Using the strengths perspective, ideally both women would have received similar interventions based on particular, individual circumstances. Operating from a non-ageist philosophy, each woman's experience would have been approached with a holistic intervention striving to connect each woman to her environment, enabling each to become a full member of her respective community.

The strengths model does not suggest that problem definitions are not taken into consideration; however, strengths do guide the course of intervention. With this model, problems are translated into needs. In keeping with its flexible nature, the model is intended for use with other forms of interventions. The key concepts focus on strengths leading to empowerment of the individual. The model literally takes the person in the environment and assists them in avoiding disenfranchisement. To maintain membership in the community it is necessary to consider, among other things, housing, financial resources, and the rules and laws that govern behavior and societal expectations.

CASE ILLUSTRATION

This case illustration takes into consideration the life cycle of two older people, Mr. and Mrs. M., married in 1936. Mr. and Mrs. M.'s marriage took place during the Great Depression. Mr. M. was a carpenter and had only seasonal work, causing frequent financial hardships for the family. Along with Mr. M.'s son from a previous marriage, the couple had two children, a daughter and a son.

Mr. M. had a long history of alcoholism that exacerbated his ill health and he retired in the early 1980s because of poor health. Because of his long history of drinking, the family experienced the typical results of such behavior, with Mrs. M. being the quintessential enabler. She did not have much of an independent life of her own but was relatively happy raising her children and enjoying her grandchildren while they were young. She had experienced mild depression for most of her married years, but never sought formal help. (She did not really recognize the depression as such.) It was only after her husband retired, her beloved sister died (her major support), her daughter moved across the country, and all of her grandchildren grew up that her depression became more pronounced. She became withdrawn, did not want to go out much, and cried a lot. Her physician prescribed an antidepressant drug in 1984 and she continued to take it until mid-1992, when she was reevaluated and the dosage and type was changed.

Person and Environment

Mrs. M. became a client at an adult day-treatment program when her son and daughter became concerned with her increased short-term memory loss. By engaging Mr. and Mrs. M. and their son and daughter in dialogue and collaboration, the practitioner gathered information about Mrs. M.'s current goodness-of-fit in her environment. The dialogue revealed that many layers of Mrs. M.'s environment were out of sync. Since Mr. M.'s retirement, the couple had been living on a fixed income (90% social security, 10% pension) that was barely adequate to meet their needs. They were able to take care of the basics, but there was very little money remaining for extras. At the time of intervention, Mr. and Mrs. M. lived in their modest home of 35 years. Since Mr. M. was a carpenter by trade, he was able to keep the home in pretty good working order, although because of his recent declining health, large jobs, such as painting and insulation, had gone unattended.

It was learned from Mr. M. that his wife couldn't seem to remember events that had occurred recently and would ask him the same question over and over within the course of a day. In speaking to Mrs. M.'s son, he stated that he had not realized how much his mother had slipped with her short-term memory until his sister, a social worker, came for a visit recently and was able to observe her mother for extended periods of time. Mrs. M.'s son had almost daily contact with his parents, and his mother was lucid when engaged in one-on-one conversations with him in person and on the telephone. He had not realized she couldn't remember their conversations.

What the practitioner was able to learn about Mrs. M.'s environment from her interaction with the family was that Mrs. M. had become increasingly more withdrawn over the past 6 months and had had very little interaction or communication with people in her environment except her husband and occasionally her son. The result was a minimal interface with other individuals and a reduced energy level. This resulted in her becoming much more dependent on her husband rather than experiencing an interdependence with him and others in her environment, leaving her coping ability greatly diminished.

Collaborative Assessment

The practitioner and case manager, Ms. Morely, from the adult day-treatment program, met with Mr. and Mrs. M. and their son and daughter. An initial assessment took place over a period of about a week. The subsequent ongoing assessment was updated as the clients' status was altered, goals changed, or new resources were required.

During the initial assessment process, which took place in the clients' home, Mr. M. could not specify what could be done for him and his wife, and Mrs. M. persistently maintained that there was nothing wrong. "We're okay," she said, "everything is just fine, if only I didn't have to worry about what we were going to eat all the time." Then she said, "Wally takes care of me." Mr. M. said that his wife didn't seem to know what to do with herself anymore, that her days pretty much went from meal to meal, going out to his shop to check up on him several times, and getting ready for bed as early as 7:30 or 8:00 P.M.

The practitioner engaged the M.s in dialogue to assist them in articulating what might be of help to them. Mr. M. said that every so often he would cook up a big batch of stew and chili and his wife would freeze it. Having the food ready seemed to relieve Mrs. M.'s anxiety about what to fix for dinner, but he said she "carried on and worried" about food anyway because she forgot about the frozen food until he reminded her. Through collaboration with the M.s about the food situation, he said he had heard about a Meals on Wheels program and thought that this service would help. He said he didn't know how to go about looking into it.

The practitioner also learned that because of Mrs. M.'s recent memory loss, her husband had been taking care of her. In addition to her antidepressant medication, she was "taking a pill for her heart," both of which Mr. M. monitored, making sure she took them at the right times. It was evident that Mr. M. cared for his wife very much; however, he was being worn down by her dependency on him and her constant stream of questions. Mr. M. said he would like his wife to get out of the house more, but he worried about her being out on her own (she liked to take walks), and furthermore, she didn't want to go any place without him.

Through this collaborative assessment the practitioner was able to see and hear many strengths in this older couple.

Mr. M. liked to cook, and Mrs. M. appreciated his effort. Mr. M. took satisfaction in helping his wife now that she was becoming forgetful. ("She nursed me through a couple of bad times, now it's my turn to take care of her.") Mr. M. had a woodworking shop in back of the house where he spent several hours a day on projects. He also loved to work in his yard. Mrs. M. liked to walk and in fact went to great lengths to tell the practitioner that these walks had been a daily part of her life for 20 years. Mrs. M. took pride in how she looked, her hair was clean and neatly done, her clothes were coordinated, and she wore make-up. Mrs. M. was very proud of both of her children and talked at length about them. Mrs. M. liked the church visitors. Mrs. M. was in good physical health. Both had supportive children.

There were other issues and needs that the clients did not identify in the initial assessment. Through further dialogue and collaboration, these issues were discussed and the practitioner helped frame them as needs. Mr. and Mrs. M. both had old, unresolved grief issues surrounding losses—the death of his son and her sister, their daughter's move across country, his failing health, her loss of memory, and inability to drive. Mr. M. was continually irritated and frustrated by his wife's memory loss. Mrs. M. felt bitterness about her "lost years" during her husband's alcoholism and resented him not supporting her with the raising of her stepson. Mrs. M. had not developed independence from Mr. M.

Informal and Formal Support Systems
Mr. and Mrs. M. had a strong informal support system. Their son and his family lived in the same town, as did Mr. M.'s brother and his wife. Included within this dynamic were three older grandchildren and next-door neighbors (husband and wife) who have always checked in on the M.s over the years to make sure "all is well." All of these people were willingly available to assist the M.s when necessary. They were also available in more routine ways, for example, for phone calls, doing errands, and stopping by to visit. The M.s' daughter was a strong support person to them even though she did not live in the same community.

At the time of the initial assessment, the M.s' community affiliations seemed to be limited. Neither of them attended church; however, there were church visitors who came by once a month, and Mrs. M. enjoyed these visits very much. The pharmacy where they obtained their medicines provided free delivery to seniors on Wednesdays and the

M.s made use of this service. There appeared to be a gap in the formal support system because the family physician was the only formal support.

Personal Program Plan

The final part of the collaborative assessment was completed in the presence of all the family members. It was agreed that Mr. M. wanted support in caring for his wife and Mrs. M. would benefit from a physical and a psychiatric evaluation. All the family members, with the exception of Mrs. M., agreed that she would benefit from the adult day-treatment program. Mrs. M.'s daughter and the practitioner explained the benefits of such a program to her mother, who said she understood but still didn't want to be away from home that long—every day from 9:00 A.M. to 3 P.M. When it became apparent that Mrs. M. would not even tour the facility, her wishes were respected. All parties involved accepted the client where she was, and at a family meeting, Mrs. M.'s decision was presented. Because Mrs. M.'s decision was respected and supported, she felt her right to self-determination and dignity was empowered and valued.

Within 24 hours Mrs. M. had a change of heart about the day program. "I don't want to go, but I know it is the best thing for me. I don't want to be like my sister who can't even remember her children's names." (Her 93-year-old sister has suffered from Alzheimer's disease for the past 10 years.)

Mr. and Mrs. M. and their children toured the day-treatment facility during the initial phase of the assessment. They were introduced to the staff and the clients who were present. They were given a tour, after which Ms. Morley explained the agency's role in the community and the case management process. Although Mrs. M. said the place looked okay to her, she didn't think she wanted to go and be with all those old people. Ms. Morley and Mrs. M.'s son explored this further with her, discussing her feelings and the meaning of embarking on this new path. The plan they all agreed upon was that Mrs. M., accompanied by her son, would come by for the next two Friday afternoons to get a better feel for what transpired there before a final decision was made. Once again, Mrs. M. felt a sense of empowerment knowing that the final decision would be hers.

A compromise was struck: Mrs. M. would only attend on Monday, Wednesday, and Friday initially. Their daughter helped her father arrange for the Meals on Wheels program, their son was able to obtain subsidized help for having the house painted and insulated.

Within a 2-week period Mr. M. was hospitalized with a serious pulmonary condition and never regained enough strength or good health to return home. He was placed in a nursing home. Mrs. M., after becoming much more depressed and confused, refused to return to the day-treatment program and was moved into her son's home. The strengths model recognizes the unforeseen dynamic nature of people-in-their-environment, characterized by instability and change, and the focus of the plan became Mrs. M. Figure 4.1 is Mrs. M.'s strengths assessment as formulated by the case manager, Mrs. M., and her son and daughter with emphasis on living arrangements.

Discussion

The strengths assessment in Figure 4.1 differs from the diagnostic assessment in that Mrs. M.'s social functioning was placed above her medical functioning. A diagnostic assessment might include the following:

> Mrs. M. is depressed over the many losses in her life; depression is psychologically based. There is no evidence of psychosis or neuro-logical disease. Mrs. M. was well groomed and polite; is physically fit, but complains of a poor appetite. Her sensory capacities are strong, and her conceptual abilities are fair. She experienced some flight of ideas; is oriented to time and place.

What emerged through the strengths assessment was a descriptive account of Mrs. M. rather than a prescriptive account. The strengths assessment, however, is supplemental and does not replace existing assessments, for example, occupational and physical therapy, as most programs adhere to an interdisciplinary approach.

Mrs. M.'s assessment highlighted the *whole* person including the six life domains with a primary focus on living arrangements as her most pressing need.

FIGURE 4.1 *Strengths Assessment*
Personal Program Plan

Social Worker/Case Manager's Name
Kate Morley

Client's Name
Mrs. M.

CURRENT SITUATION: WHAT'S GOING ON NOW?	PERSONAL GOALS: WHAT I'D LIKE TO HAVE/ACHIEVE	RESOURCES: INTERNAL/EXTERNAL WHAT HAVE I USED? WHAT CAN I USE?	PRIORITIZED NEEDS/WANTS: WHAT STEPS DO I TAKE?
Living Arrangements: My living situation...			
currently lives with son and his wife in a three story house; has a room on the main floor next to the bath	plans to return home	used to organize her day around household chores and family members; help out daughter-in-law with chores; used to enjoy early morning alone time	wants to return home; wants to maintain contact with family and friends; wants to remain independent; wants to feel ok about living with son
Social Supports: Who's important in my life/where can I go for support?			
making adjustments to new living situation; spends alone time on personal reflection; minimal community involvement (i.e., church clubs)	wants more contact with sister-in-law; wants to develop friendships; wants contact with daughter; wants contact with other family members	used to go to church; used to visit friends and family members; used to work in garden; used to read daily scriptures; used to call and write to daughter	will go on weekly outings with sister-in-law; will attend day-treatment program and make friends; will call daughter; will go to church

Social Worker/Case Manager's Name
Kate Morley

Client's Name
Mrs. M.

CURRENT SITUATION: WHAT'S GOING ON NOW?	PERSONAL GOALS: WHAT I'D LIKE TO HAVE/ACHIEVE	RESOURCES: INTERNAL/EXTERNAL WHAT HAVE I USED? WHAT CAN I USE?	PRIORITIZED NEEDS/WANTS: WHAT STEPS DO I TAKE?
Relationships: How do I feel about my relationships with others (interpersonal) and my relationship with myself (intrapersonal)?			
feels lonely and misses husband	wants to work on blending in to new living arrangement (be separate and together)	used to go over to sister-in-law's	same as above; and,
feels like she's imposing on son	wishes she still had her sister	used to travel to visit daughter	wants more interaction with others
minimal contact with family and friends		used to visit (over fence) with neighbors	wants family to "let her be" (independence)
is sociable			reminisce (grief work) about sister
Personal Care: What activities can I do to care for myself or others?			
takes care of all her personal needs	keep walking	health conscious	keep walking
takes pride in how she looks	get permanent and hair cut	watches weight	keep watching weight
always clean and neat looking		walks daily	make hair appointment
		used to polish nails	
Education: What would I like to learn?			
is conversant	do a little more reading	used to read books, newspapers, and scripture	read daily scriptures
is content with who she is now		used to experiment with and adapt recipes	

Social Worker/Case Manager's Name
Kate Morley

Client's Name
Mrs. M.

CURRENT SITUATION: WHAT'S GOING ON NOW?	PERSONAL GOALS: WHAT I'D LIKE TO HAVE/ACHIEVE	RESOURCES: INTERNAL/EXTERNAL WHAT HAVE I USED? WHAT CAN I USE?	PRIORITIZED NEEDS/WANTS: WHAT STEPS DO I TAKE?

Leisure/Recreation: What activities do I like/how do I spend my time?

goes to church on Sunday A.M.	would like to travel a bit	used to crochet	take trips with son and daughter
works jigsaw puzzles	likes to sit by herself and	used to play cards (loved solitaire)	go visit daughter
goes shopping and to lunch	reflect	used to work in garden	try crocheting again
with sister-in-law			"Be Quiet"

Health: How do I stay physically and mentally healthy?

physical health excellent	attend day-treatment	always have a daily walk	wants to keep going to
sight and hearing excellent	program daily	has always enjoyed good health	day-treatment program
sleeps well	keep walking		wants to walk each day alone
eats well	take medicine regularly		drink less coffee (or change
exercises (walks)			to decaf)

Financial: What's my money situation?

receives social security	wants to understand	used to "tuck" money away	will go over financial records
($320/mo)	financial situation better:	received small inheritance	with son
medicare insurance	"My husband use to take	(long gone)	
small savings	care of everything."		
son and daughter assist when			
needed			

Personal Strengths List

What do I like about myself? __weight, agility (they call her spry at day program), looks, friendliness__

What are my strengths? __good health, like people, get on well with people__

What assets do others think I have? __friendly, supportive, kindhearted__

The preceding assessment plan was based upon the four dimensions described in Chapter 3: (a) A client's current status—Mrs. M. could no longer live solely alone and alternatives were sought; (b) stated personal goals—Mrs. M. wanted to maintain her independence and "not be a burden" on her son and daughter-in-law; (c) internal and external resources—Mrs. M. set about doing chores to help out her daughter-in-law even though she said she felt like she was an intruder, and she called her old church to ask if they would come to visit her at her son's home; (d) priority of needs—Mrs. M. needed a safe, secure environment in which to live, a supportive family, and hope that she might be able to return home.

In the process necessary to formulate this plan, the case manager and Mrs. M. began building a working, trusting relationship. Mrs. M. said that when Ms. Morley asked her to "tell me what living alone means to you, and what kinds of things you can do so that might happen," she felt listened to for the first time since she had left her home. This was a first step in her challenging, new life situation and the beginning of her feeling empowered. Mrs. M.'s problems were being translated into needs.

PROBLEMS	NEEDS
1. Husband no longer at home to care for her	A safe, secure living environment
2. Leaving home of 35 years	Explore avenues for more independence
3. Mrs. M. feels like a burden to her son and daughter-in-law	Seek ways to fit in without feeling like an intruder (i.e., help with chores)

By starting where the client was and proceeding at Mrs. M.'s pace, an adult-to-adult relationship began to unfold that was based upon healthy communication and set the tone for future dialogues. By conducting the assessment in the home, Mrs. M. felt comfortable and less threatened by what was taking place. This in-home assessment was also advantageous for the case manager as she was able to gain valuable insight into how Mrs. M. functioned in her daily routine. Throughout the initial assessment, Ms. Morley continually emphasized Mrs. M.'s strengths. Mrs. M. was surprised as she repeatedly made reference to her problems, declaring that she couldn't think of many strengths to help her through this one. This shock lessened for Mrs. M., however, as she gained trust in Ms. Morley, who continued to reframe the problems into wants and needs.

For example, one interaction occurred as follows. "Now that my husband is gone I just don't know what to do with myself, it seems like I have nothing but problems ahead of me." Ms. Morley replied, "Let's make a list of all the things you have to do in the next couple of days." This pleased Mrs. M. and she began her list: (a) get groceries ("But this is a problem because I don't drive anymore.") (b) go to the day-treatment program ("But this is a problem because I feel like I need to stay by the phone.") (c) think about moving in with my son ("But this is a problem because I don't want to be a burden, and besides, what would I do with the house and all this stuff?"). Ms. Morley reminded Mrs. M. that there was ample food in the freezer and that she would still be receiving Meals on Wheels, that there was a telephone at the day treatment program through which she could receive messages about her husband, and that Mrs. M. and the social worker could arrange a time when they could meet with Mrs. M.'s son and his wife to explore the pending move. This dialogue seemed to cheer Mrs. M. a bit, and she said, "Gosh, I think I feel a little better, maybe I can make it through this, but I really do miss Wally." Ms. Morley then asked Mrs. M. if she felt ready to return to the day-treatment program, and she replied, "I'm not sure, let me think about it." Ms. Morely said, "Tell me what makes you feel uncertain." This last interchange put Mrs. M. in control, and made her the expert in her decision.

Mrs. M.'s strengths assessment was an ongoing process and there were updates reflecting her accomplishments and changing needs throughout her time in the program.

Assessing Individual Strengths and Supports
Life strengths and supports are not fixed, nor can they be evaluated once and then used as an ongoing standard. Life strengths shift and sway as part of an overall picture, forever changing (Kivnick, 1993).

Recognizing and defining client strengths is central to collaborative assessment; however, it is often difficult for clients to see their own strengths clearly. The following are some questions that can be used to encourage clients to talk about strengths set forth by Kivnick (1993):

What is it in your life that gives you hope?

What is your religious affiliation?

How do you like to express your religious beliefs?

What is it in your life that gives you a sense of security?

What part of your life is it most important that *you* stay in charge of?

What kinds of independence would you find especially painful to give up?

What is it that has always given you confidence in yourself?

What kinds of things do you enjoy doing…activities?

What kinds of things have you always been good at?

What kinds of things are you good at now?

Who is important to you in your life today? Where are they?

Can you tell me about…your best friend?…your marriage?

What is there about your life that you wish had been different?

What has been most meaningful about your life so far?

What is it about your life today that…makes you feel most alive?…is most worth living?…makes you feel most like yourself?

Adapted from "Everyday Mental Health: A Guide to Assessing Life Strengths," *Generations*, 17 (1), 18–19.

The case manager's knowledge of client strengths becomes invaluable in helping to construct the possibility of change, transformation, and hope. Figure 4.2 shows Mrs. M.'s individual personal program plan building on identified strengths.

A personal program plan is developed by the case manager and all other involved parties based upon one life domain at a time. The focus is on the client's set of prioritized needs within that life domain. There are no given guidelines for completion, and the direction, complexity, or simplicity of the plan is based upon the client's individual needs. The personal program plan is updated with each client contact. Additional action steps can be added as needed. This can be done weekly or monthly. There can be several personal program plans in effect at one time based upon the client's needs, and one or more of the top priority needs worked on from several life domains.

In the case of Mrs. M., only one plan, living arrangements, was being worked on for the time being. Present when this personal program plan was made were Mrs. M., her son and his wife, the physician, and Ms. Morley, the case manager.

Mrs. M. had experienced a rapid sequence of events that forced her to be abruptly moved from her home and she was having a difficult time adjusting. When she first arrived at her son's home she was disoriented and would repack her bags daily and announce that she was ready to return home. Ms. Morley and the son spent time talking to Mrs. M. about the necessity for the move, and they all discussed possible alternatives. One alternative that they explored was placement in a retirement community where Mrs. M. could live with some degree of independence; the other was to move into the apartment in the downstairs of her son's home. Mrs. M. was adamant, however, about wanting to return home, so this return became her long-term goal. The long-term goal was listed even though the team at the day-treatment program and Mrs. M.'s son thought that returning home to live alone was improbable. Just as the practitioner and Mrs. M.'s family had supported her in not wanting to enter the day-treatment program, they now respected her wish to return home.

The short-term goal for Mrs. M. is a restatement of the prioritized needs from the strengths assessment:

Wants to return home

Wants to maintain contact with family and friends

Wants to remain independent

Wants to feel okay about living with son, temporarily

FIGURE 4.2   *Personal Program Plan*

Social Worker/Case Manager's Name   Client's Name
  Kate Morley   Mrs. M.

Life Domain: x Living Arrangements   __ Social Supports   __ Personal Care
                  __ Education   __ Leisure/Recreational   __ Financial
                                               __ Relationships
                                               __ Health

Long-term Goal: To return home; however, all parties agreed that this may take some time and in the meantime Mrs. M. and her son and
                  daughter-in-law would concentrate on the adjustments necessary to make Mrs. M.'s transition a pleasant one.

MEASURABLE SHORT-TERM TREATMENT GOALS AND INTERMEDIATE ACTION STEPS	RESPONSIBILITY FOR ACTION PLAN: PROVIDER NAME, LICENSE INITIALS; FREQUENCY; MODALITY; REFERRALS	DATE TO BE ACCOMPLISHED	DATE COMPLETED
Mrs. M. wants to work on "blending" into new living arrangements. She wants her son and his family not to treat her preferentially and for them to carry on with their own lives. She wants to have some autonomy.	Mrs. M., her son, and daughter-in-law	6/30/92	6/30/92
Mrs. M. will keep her room in order, will load and unload the dishwasher, will dust furniture on Fridays.	Mrs. M.	daily	ongoing
Mrs. M. will go on an outing on Saturdays with sister-in-law.	Mrs. M. and sister-in-law.	6/4, 11, 18, 25	6/30

Mrs. M. will begin investigating alternative   son, Mrs. Morley (CM)   6/30   6/30
living situations.

If more than one page, signatures are required on the last page and are optional on the other pages

Client's Signature
    Mrs. M.
Date___June 1, 1992
Social Worker's Signature
    K. Morley, CM
Date___June 1, 1992

Signature and title (other)
    D.M.   son
Date___June 1, 1992
Signature and title (other)
    Dr. Dearheart
Date___June 1, 1992

Mrs. M.'s biggest fear was that she was a burden on her son and his wife, despite their repeated reassurances to the contrary. Mrs. M. said that if she were a daughter-in-law she wouldn't have wanted her mother-in-law to move in with them. Mrs. M. and her daughter-in-law had ongoing dialogue about this. Mrs. M.'s daughter-in-law assured Mrs. M. that she was nothing like her own mother-in-law. Mrs. M.'s daughter-in-law stated, in fact, that "you have been a wonderful mother-in-law, and having you live with us is our way of paying you back." This was highlighted as a strength of Mrs. M.'s—the care and concern she has shown for her children over the years. This put Mrs. M. at ease, but she needed constant reassurance during the first months. The case manager asked Mrs. M. what might make the transition a little easier. Mrs. M. replied, "Maybe if I had something to do." It was agreed that Mrs. M. would have responsibilities for some chores around the house. This was another of Mrs. M.'s highlighted strengths—her ability to organize her time around household chores and meals.

As shown on the personal program plan, the action steps are measurable and incremental and include tasks that the client can easily accomplish, starting with "where the client is" and what she can do. With Mrs. M.'s wants in mind, the process of achieving her wishes through actions had begun. Happily, albeit reluctantly, Mrs. M. flashed a smile after they had completed the plan and said, "Now, let's get to work!"

Evaluation

With these measurable action steps, Mrs. M. started to feel a sense of community and membership with her son, his wife, and her sister-in-

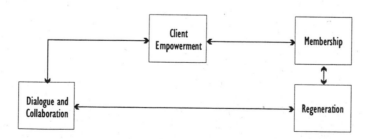

FIGURE 4.3 *Mrs. M.'s process of empowerment*

law and took more pleasure in the Saturday outings. The regeneration that occurred as a result of this personal program plan became one of the pieces that helped Mrs. M. with the transition associated with her relocation. Her progress through the strengths assessment could be mapped as shown in Figure 4.3.

At the end of the agreed upon date for accomplishment of Mrs. M.'s goals, all parties met again to discuss the process and progress, and began a new personal program plan. Mrs. M. decided that she wanted to work on the life domain of social supports for her next plan. The personal program plan was developed in the home.

Summary

The focus for both the strengths assessment and the personal program plan has been on living, on dynamic interactions, and active participation in the environment. Through these means, the client is assisted in reviewing, renewing, and reworking a life that may have otherwise become static.

For Mrs. M. in the example and other older adults, old age presents new challenges. Through the strengths model, they relearn how to access existing capacities to manage day-to-day needs. Mental health can hang in the balance as older people face the daily challenges of survival. According to Kivnick (1993)

> Throughout the life cycle, everyday mental health may be described as an attempt to live meaningfully, in a particular set of social and environmental circumstances, relying on a particular collection of resources and supports. Simply said, we all try to do the best we can with what we have. (p. 15)

By respecting Mrs. M. as her own person and recognizing her strengths, the strengths model enabled Mrs. M. to develop resources and supports to help her live a meaningful life in her new environment.

REFERENCES

Butler, R., Lewis, M., & Sunderland, T. (1991). *Aging and mental health: Positive psychosocial and biomedical approaches* (4th ed.). New York: Merrill Publishing Co.

George, L. (1993, Winter/Spring). Depressive disorders and symptoms in later life. *Generations, 17*(1), 35–38.

Glick, I., Weiss, R., & Parkes, C.M. (1974). *The first year of bereavement.* New York: John Wiley & Sons.

Greenwald, B. S., & Kramer-Ginsberg, E. (1988). Age at onset in geriatric depression: Relationship to clinical variables. *Journal of Affective Disorders, 15*, 61–68.

Gurland, B. J., Dean, L., Cross, P., & Golden, R. (1980). The epidemiology of depression and dementia in the elderly: The use of multiple indicators of these conditions. In J. O. Cole & J. E. Barrett (Eds.), *Psychopathology of the aged.* New York: Raven Press, 72–98.

Hooyman, N. R., & Kiyak, H. A. (1991). *Social gerontology: A multidisciplinary perspective* (2nd ed.). Boston: Allyn and Bacon.

Hunt, M. (1991). Blue skies ahead: New medications and specialized psychotherapy are curing the depressed elderly. *American Health, 10*, 53.

Kermis, M. (1986). *Mental health in late life.* Boston: Janes & Bartlett.

Kivnick, H. Q. (1993). Everyday mental health: A guide to assessing life strengths. *Generations, 17*(1), 13–20.

Klerman, G. L., Lavori, P. W., Rice, J., Reich, T., Endicott, J., Andreasen, N. C., Keller, M. B., & Hirschfield, R. M. A. (1985). Birth-cohort trends in rates of major depression disorders among relatives of patients with affective disorder. *Archives of General Psychiatry, 42*, 689–693.

Miller, M. (1979). *Suicide after sixty: The final alternative.* New York: Springer Publishing Co.

National Institutes of Health. (1992). *Diagnosis and treatment of depression late in life.* Washington, DC: U.S. Government Printing Office.

Neurol, A. (1991). Memory complaints in older adults: Fact or fiction? *Journal of the American Medical Association, 266*, 1070–1071.

Osgood, N. J. (1985). *Suicide and the elderly: A practitioner's guide to diagnosis and mental health intervention.* Rockville, MD: Aspen Publishers.

Parkes, C. M. (1965). Bereavement and mental illness. *British Journal of Medical Psychiatry, 37*(6), 1–26.

Ruegg, R G., Zisook, S., & Swerdlow, N. R. (1988). Depression in the aged: An overview. *Psychiatric Clinics of North America, 11*, 83–99.

Seligman, M. E. P. (1975). *Helplessness.* San Francisco: W.H. Freeman.

Weiss, R. S. (Ed.). (1973). *Loneliness: The experience of emotional and social isolation.* Cambridge, MA: MIT Press.

CHAPTER FIVE

Suicide and Older Adults

THIS CHAPTER DISCUSSES SUICIDE and the application of the strengths model of practice as a means of suicide prevention for older adults. There is an overview of suicide among older adults, discussion of the impact of ageism on suicide rates, and a look at risks. With this information as a backdrop, the strengths model is used to reframe service intervention with suicidal older adults.

The Environment, Age, and Suicide

Suicide is the eighth leading cause of death in the United States and accounts for over thirty thousand deaths each year. Among the general population, the suicide rate was recorded as 12.4 per 100,000 persons in 1992. However, the suicide rate of older people was higher than in the general population, with a rate of 20.5 per 100,000. Persons 65 and older make up 12.5% of the population and account for 20.9% of suicides annually. By contrast, young people between the ages of 15 and 24 account for 14.8% of the population and account for 15.8% of the suicides annually. Since statistics on suicide rates were first collected in 1900, the highest rates recorded to date (35 to 40 per 100,000) occurred during and immediately following the Great Depression of the early 1930s. Since the mid-1940s, suicide rates among the elderly declined significantly until an upward trend appeared between 1981 and 1987. During that time span, suicide rates among the older persons increased from 17 to 20 per 100,000. Suicide rates have also increased among older African American males, but at a considerably lower rate of 15 suicides per 100,000 (McIntosh, 1992). See Figure 5.1.

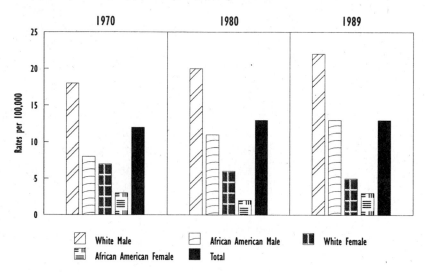

(a) Suicide Rates by Gender and Race

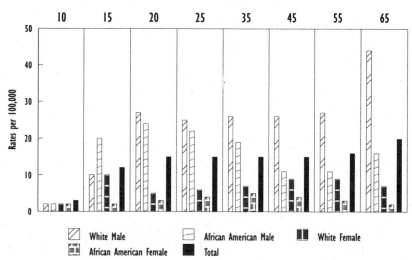

(b) Suicide Rates by Age

FIGURE 5.1 *(a) Suicide rates by gender and race, and (b) Suicide rates by age*

Data from "Epidemiology of Suicide in the Elderly," by J. L. McIntosh, 1992, *Suicide and Life-Threatening Behavior, 22* (1), 15–35.

Among older men, the risk of suicide increases with age, accounting for rates three times higher than for the general population (McIntosh, 1992). Among women, suicide statistics have remained relatively low. Rates of death by suicide among older women are 6.6 per 100,000, considerably lower than for older males. Traditionally, women are at greatest risk of suicide during midlife, with a significant decline in risk occurring thereafter (Manton, Blazer, & Woodbury, 1987). Although there is no definitive explanation for the significant difference in the rate of suicide among older men and women, some research strongly suggests that differences in coping skills reflect sex role differences and patterns of socialization (Canetto, 1992).

DETERIORATING ENVIRONMENT

Among the many myths about the older adults is that they are somehow justified in their desire to contemplate or commit suicide. Despite the physical decrements that accompany the aging process, changes in appearance, and increasing dependency, there are many positive aspects to growing old. For example, older persons have more leisure time, time-tested coping skills, and life experiences in a variety of settings. Death by suicide need not be the last choice for those who feel lost and alone in late life. Identifying and embracing the strengths acquired throughout life can give older people hope for the future.

Take the case of an older stroke victim. Mr. Dancer, age 72, lived alone in a second floor apartment in a run-down section of town. He was a widower of 18 months, had two children, one of whom lived in a nearby community, and an older brother who lived across town. Mr. Dancer suffered a stroke and had been in a wheelchair for three months. He was unable to return to work and was having financial problems. His apartment was not wheelchair accessible, he spent most days in bed, refused to work with therapists, did not answer his phone, and became isolated from his family and the community.

On a routine home visit, the home health nurse found Mr. Dancer in bed with all the shades drawn. He was depressed and said he could see no reason to go on living. "I can't even get to the kitchen to cook anymore. What's the use anyway, since Emma's gone, not much seems to matter." The nurse referred Mr. Dancer to social services and the social worker went to his home to perform an assessment. In the dialogue during the initial interview, the social worker discovered that Mr. Dancer's wife had died after a long illness that left him with a heavy financial burden. He subsequently sold the family home in order to pay off the hospital bill. He sold most of the household furniture, found a new home for his dog, and moved into his current apartment. He said his daughter wanted him to live with her. "Hell, I'm not going to burden her with a lame old man. She's young and has a busy life for herself." She calls me all the time, but I don't have nothing to say. What's to tell…I miss her mother? That would just make her feel sad." The worker also learned that Mr. Dancer's brother came by at least once a week and brought him food and checked on him. "I appreciate Joe coming by, but he's getting up there in years, and besides he has a sick wife to take of. He doesn't need me to pull on him too." Although Mr. Dancer was clearly despondent, the social worker received a couple of clues that he might want to get out of bed. Another meeting was scheduled for the next morning. Mr. Dancer reluctantly agreed to invite his daughter and brother to attend.

In the majority of cases, suicide among older adults can be prevented. Mental health practitioners continue to conduct research and explore creative ways to work with aged individuals and their systems of support. The strengths model of practice includes an array of techniques that enhances the older person's ability to assess and adapt or change the conditions that can lead to suicidal ideation. Many of the resources required for this shift of thinking and actions are found within older people themselves. Thus the strengths model recognizes that older adults can offset their potential suicidal risks by focusing on strengths.

In the case of Mr. Dancer, the social worker helped him identify several strengths: (a) caring and consideration for his daughter and brother, (b) compassion and concern for the dog he had placed in an adoptive home, (c) passion about cooking, and (d) a keen eye for food presentation. Mr. Dancer was surprised when the worker recited some of his perceived strengths. "I've been feeling so down and sorry for myself lately, I hardly recognize the person you're talking about. How'd you figure it out?"

The first strength, caring for his family, was easy to discern from their discussions. She reminded him that when he told her about his dog, he got tears in his eyes and said, "Damn, I never thought I'd miss the little rascal so much." When he talked about his cooking, his eyes lit up. Also he showed her some pictures of the food he had cooked and served for various occasions. The social worker also noticed when she went into the kitchen that his cooking utensils had been retained and were readily visible.

As a result of this dialogue, Mr. Dancer was able to identify other strengths. He said he was a good poker player and expressed a possible interest in calling old poker pals. He also mentioned a class he took in French baking and that he had received top marks. The next step was to prepare a plan of action with Mr. Dancer.

Characteristics of Suicide: Relationship to Environment

Among the factors that contribute to senior suicide are marital status, social class, occupation, and the living environment. Regardless of age, suicide rates have historically been higher for nonmarried persons than married persons (Durkheim, 1987/1951; Kastenbaum & Aisenberg, 1972). Many researchers suggest a relationship between retirement and suicide (c.f. Butler, 1975; Kopell, 1977; Miller, 1979; Sainsbury, 1968; Wolff, 1971). For older persons living in urban areas, suicide rates are high, especially those in lower socioeconomic, inner-city neighborhoods (Gardner, Bahn, & Mack, 1964; Henery & Short, 1954). Moving and fear of institutionalization and dependency are factors related to suicide among the older adults (Miller, 1979), as are isolation, desolation, and loneliness.

While none of the above factors are to be diminished as explanations for senior suicide, it should be noted that the more recent findings from psychological autopsies (the psychological correlate of the medical autopsy) have contradicted some of the more popularly held beliefs about older adult suicides. For example, over one-third of the senior suicide victims in Clark's (1991) and Conwell, Rotenberg, and Caine's (1990) studies were married at the time of death, more than half lived with someone, either a spouse or family member, with the majority having a variety of social contacts inside and outside the home. Furthermore, major life stressors were no more prevalent among older suicide victims just prior to their death than were true for most other older persons. Findings showed that only 11% were faced with a change in their living situations, only 7% had lost a spouse by death within the last year, and only 5% experienced any sort of financial hardship. There was, however, a relationship between major depressive conditions and death by suicide (Clark, 1991; Conwell, Rotenberg, & Caine, 1990). One explanation for these contradictions could be that as societal and personal conditions change for older adults in our society, so do the circumstances surrounding their reasons for suicide. For mental health practitioners this implies a heightened challenge as well as continued vigilance in considering the many varied risks involved, leaving no stone unturned when assessing suicide among older persons.

Social, Economic, and Political Perspectives

Suicide among older adults has not been sufficiently addressed by our society. Clark (1992) goes so far as to declare it a major public health problem that begs for social and political intervention. The obvious question is "Why have senior suicides been left unattended?" Partial answers can be found in rampant ageism and prevailing stereotypes, but we also have to look at what it means to be old in America.

Comfort (1976) stated that "the real curse of being old is the ejection from a citizenship traditionally based on work...a demeaning idleness, nonuse, not being called on any longer to contribute, and hence being put down as a spent person of no public account" (p. 16). This curse ascribes the status of a nonperson to older people, who are rendered arbitrarily roleless. To a large degree, older people today are left to define their own roles in society. Quality of life frequently enters into how that role is defined. To enjoy what would be considered a healthy old age certain ingredients are necessary: affordable medical care, decent housing, recreation, some measure of good physical and emotional health, formal and informal supports, and adequate finances. Unfortunately, not all of these ingredients exist for all older people.

Looking at politics from the infrastructure perspective, it would appear that there need to be more flexible retirement options, more available public housing, and reform of the health care system. Clark (1992) cites other policies that affect suicide among the older adults: "growing popular sympathy for euthanasia, physician-assisted suicide, and 'death-with-dignity' legislation—hand-in-hand with diminishing public awareness of potential dangers and abuses posed."

The reason that suicide rates continue to be high in the aged population may be explained by the suicide risk factors cited above. As displayed in Figure 5.2, one of the most significant factors is loss of a spouse, children, friends, job, health, self-esteem, etc., and the subsequent isolation that follows. These multiple losses can leave many older people with unresolved feelings of profound sadness, detachment, and loneliness. Any one of these factors, or any combination, can lead to

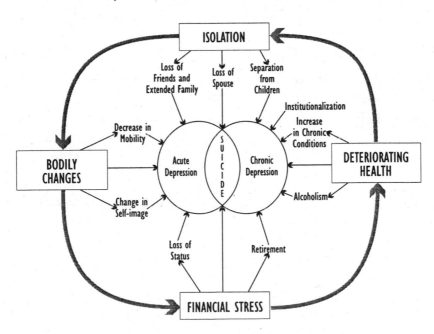

FIGURE 5.2 *Factors leading to suicide in older adults*

acute or chronic depression. Risks are discussed further in the section on assessments.

In the case of Mr. Dancer, at least nine of the risk factors seen in Figure 5.2 applied: loss of spouse, loss of friends, isolation, decreased mobility, bodily changes, loss of status, financial stress, deteriorating health, and acute depression. Through continued dialogue and collaboration, the social worker and Mr. Dancer made a list of these losses, opening the way to talk more openly about his feelings regarding recent losses that had befallen him. Talking about his losses and how they affected him instilled hope for Mr. Dancer and the beginning of a sense of empowerment.

Underreporting

The statistics on senior suicide, as they stand, are alarmingly high. One shudders at what the true numbers might be when underreporting is taken into consideration. Butler, Lewis, and Sunderland (1991) noted that "the actual rate of suicide is underreported because of shame and guilt. Some religious groups such as Catholics and Orthodox Jews have denied burial rites to persons who completed suicide. It is also underestimated because of deception to protect life insurance benefits" (p. 129). Other factors contributing to underreporting could be the fact that older persons usually suffer from chronic conditions, are under treatment and on medication, and are chronologically closer to death. Suicide is often disguised as overdosing on medications (which goes without notice), ceasing to take medications, or involvement in fatal accidents. Taking these medical factors into account, family members might be embarrassed to have the death of a loved one reported as a suicide. Consequently, some families request the cause of death be reported as natural or as related to a specific medical condition (Blazer, Bachar, & Manton, 1986). Sometimes the family wishes are honored but often they are entirely ignored.

Methods

Examples of nonviolent methods of suicide are overdosing, poisoning, and carbon monoxide asphyxiation. Violent methods used to complete suicide are guns, hanging, immolation (setting self on fire), and jumping from high places. The use of firearms as a method ranks highest among seniors, second, hanging, and gas and solid or liquid poisons account for the majority of remaining senior suicides (McIntosh & Santos, 1985–86).

TRADITIONAL INTERVENTIONS

Some of the traditional methods of intervention are briefly summarized in this section. They include group therapy, reminiscence and life therapy, and creative therapies such as art, music, and dance. Group therapy is an intervention for the older adult client that can be used in such settings as nursing homes, private outpatient programs, housing projects, and mental health facilities (Osgood, 1985). Groups are especially effective for seniors who are vulnerable to loneliness, stress, physical or emotional challenges, and suicide.

There are many advantages to groups for older adults. The group provides the opportunity to confront feelings of alienation by open expression of feelings. Members can learn from each other and share information, can learn and practice interpersonal skills, and can offer hope through sharing successes (Yalom, 1985). Specific types of support groups that work well with older adults are reality orientation, life review/reminiscence, remotivation, and psychotherapy.

Life review/reminiscence for a time was not popularly supported. It was thought of as excessive dwelling on remote memories, as a result of loss of recent memory or even evidence of senility (Butler, et al., 1991; Sherman, 1991). This is no longer the case, however, and reminiscence is viewed as part of the normal life process so crucial to the emotional livelihood of an older person. For an older person, reminiscence helps to resolve past conflicts, thus establishing the development of a coherent life history (Butler, et al., 1991). Also, it serves to highlight the skills and coping mechanisms people used to proceed through crises in their lives and regain a sense of control over their situations.

In reviewing clients' personal histories with them, social workers can help clients to see the many strengths and skills that they have used to resolve a lifetime of difficult situations. By understanding that they may still be able to use many of these skills, older clients can be empowered to face the future with greater confidence.

Life review for older people suffering from depression is a necessary and healthy process and a useful tool for the maintenance of mental health (Butler, et al., 1991). In the context of the strengths perspective of practice, life review leads to a process of dialogue and collaboration between the client and the practitioner. This ability to understand clients on their own terms and as persons embedded in their unique life histories is a prerequisite to engaging them in dialogue.

There are several creative therapies that are used when working with vulnerable older adults. Using the various arts—music, visual art, drama, dance—is naturally therapeutic, allowing creative expression such as development of personal insight, and self-awareness. It expands the consciousness and helps the individual to become more aware of self in a natural way by emphasizing the connection between mind and body (Osgood, 1975). Other creative therapies that are growing in popularity and usefulness are animal therapy and horticultural therapy.

Attitudes on Aging

Older people reach old age because they have survived, many times against great odds. The suicide rate among old people *is* high; however, it cannot be disputed that their survival into old age suggests that their viability and allegiance to life should not be underestimated (Kastenbaum, 1992) or devalued when seeking appropriate intervention strategies for older adults who are suicidal.

Lay people and professionals must avoid the rigid application of stereotyped assumptions about old people, specifically that growing old, illness, and the prospect of dying somehow offer protection from a high lethality or suicidality orientation (Kastenbaum, 1992). Ageism rears its ugly head all too often in our society and serves to reinforce these and other stereotypes about older persons.

Ageism

The failure to look at old age through clear, unobscured lenses does not have to do with aging as much as ageism. Aging is a real process that eventually affects all individuals, whereas ageism is a constriction in perception and thought that rearranges power relations and is like other forms of discrimination or prejudice. When aging, people may gain or lose parts of themselves; however, with ageism people are shaped into something that is always less (Cooper, 1986; Perkins, 1992). The most important aspect of ageism that affects suicide among older adults is ageism among professionals. In spite of the ever-increasing need for mental health services and interventions, aged individuals are grossly underserved by the mental health profession. This is due in part to what Butler, et al. (1991) called negative countertransference whereby mental health personnel react to older persons in inappropriate ways that are reminiscent of previous patterns of relating to parents and other key childhood figures. Not only do mental health personnel need to deal with leftover feelings from their pasts, they must also be aware of a multitude of negative cultural attitudes about older persons (Butler, et al., 1991).

The prevailing belief is that it is futile to address the psychological aspects of the aged because older people are rigid and cannot change, because they lack the necessary energy for intervention, or because they are near death and do not need the attention (why bother?). Often there is a distortion by service providers in their understanding of why a specific instance of suicide has occurred, leading them to believe it is a rational suicide or a psychologically sound person's right to die. A strong cultural bias creeps in and the forces and motives implicated in cases of suicide by the aged individual are overlooked (Butler, 1975; Richardson, Lowenstein, & Weissberg, 1989). The views expressed above are an example of suspension of belief, where practitioners either buy into entrenched stereotypes or assume that the client's views come from faulty perceptions. With the strengths model there is a shift to the practitioner's suspension of disbelief, which encourages the emergence of the truth from the client and which could result in preventing the suicide.

In the case of Mr. Dancer, after two frustrating sessions early on with the client, the social worker found that she had to suspend the beliefs she held about older people's lack of resiliency and inability to change late in life. Some countertransference issues emerged that had to be dealt with. Several years before, the social worker's father had experienced late-life depression and had stubbornly refused professional help, which resulted in a lengthy hospitalization. This countertransference was resolved by ongoing dialogue with the supervisor about the unfinished business regarding the social worker and her father. The process of dialoguing with the supervisor aided the worker *and* Mr. Dancer to begin, in earnest, a dialogue and collaboration of their own. This early-stage dialogue allowed Mr. Dancer to become more focused on his losses and the worker was able to accept the client "where he was": frightened, alone, and depressed, with no desire to go on with his life. Using the concepts of the strengths model, Mr. Dancer's progress to date could be mapped as shown in Figure 5.3.

THEORETICAL CONCEPTS AND ENVIRONMENTAL INFLUENCES

Researchers in disciplines such as sociology, psychology, social work, and suicidology continue to search for answers to suicide. Table 5.1 outlines the predominate theories guiding the study of suicide, lists components of each theory, and lists the subsequent function that emanates from the theory. Suicide risk is then rated as low, moderate, or high in accordance with the function.

The following is a brief historical overview highlighting two of the theoretical concepts applied to the study of suicide among older adults. Durkheim's (1897/1951) studies of suicide were formative and have shed much light on the phenomenon of suicide. It was his view that suicide rates are higher in more modern societies largely because of more individuation of members, division of labor, and specialization of

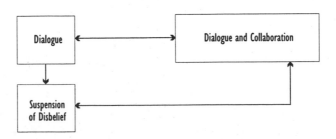

FIGURE 5.3 *Mr. Dancer's progress*

TABLE 5.1 *Comparative Analysis of Sociological and Psychological Theories of Suicide Relate to Older Adults*

MAJOR THEORIES	COMPONENTS	FUNCTION	SUICIDE RISK
Sociological	value on age	age viewed as pathway to wisdom	low
	integration within society/community	collective forces of society and community restrains suicide, constant interchange among members, shared energy and mutual support	low
	overdependence within society/ community	leads to inability to function on one's own	low
	with aging, moral force recedes	as older person withdraws, support for both goals or commitment diminishes	low to moderate
	less integration within society/ community	no mutual support	moderate
	modern societies	individuation of members, division of labor, extended families dissipated, high value placed on productivity	high
	integration weakens with loss of roles	major role losses include family, work, work-related functions, and organizations	high (egoistic suicide)
Psychological	terminal illness	older person comes to accept life on any terms	low
	physical illness	could be a factor, however, not as predominate as once believed	moderate to low
	loss of status within society and community	loss is systematic, resources diminish, judged on age not performance	moderate to low (anomic suicide)

continued next page

TABLE 5.1, *continued*

MAJOR THEORIES	COMPONENTS	FUNCTION	SUICIDE RISK
	intolerable despair	induces discouragement and inability to see tolerable path to meaningful life	moderate to high
	season of losses	losses include emotional, social, psychological, financial, spouse, children, friends, self-esteem, personal control, competence, hearing, sight, physical health, mobility, job, etc.	high
	depression	profound, painful rejection resulting in loss of interest in life	high
	loss exacerbates depression	loss of loved ones contributes to depression, life becomes empty and meaningless	high
	helplessness	as roles and status change, older person feels loss of control of life	high

tasks. Others before him (c.f. Morselli, 1882/1979) and after (c.f. Quinney, 1965; Lynn, 1969) have arrived at similar conclusions.

In societies where there is a high value placed on the aged, suicide rates for older adults are lower. For example, rates for Native Indian men in Canada approach zero when these men reach old age. As cultures have become more developed and diversified, however, age is no longer viewed as a pathway to wisdom, extended families become dissipated, people are seen as interchangeable and dispensable, and progress and productivity is more highly valued than any individual person. With this script orchestrating progressive times, senior suicide rates have risen (Seiden, 1983).

From the sociological perspective, Durkheim (1897/1951) emphasized the importance of integration or belonging within a society. It was

Durkheim's belief that suicide cannot be explained by psychological or biological factors alone, but rather it is the nature and extent of one's involvement in society that is the decisive factor in suicide. Furthermore, he contended that individuals have little or no control over various social factors within the society and that these factors also influence suicide rates. In a cohesive society there is a constant interchange of ideas and feelings between its members that resembles mutual moral support, a collective, shared energy that does not ask individuals to rely solely upon their own resources. The less individuals are integrated into society, the more vulnerable they are to suicide. A caveat exists, however, in that excessive integration, or overdependence on society, can also lead to suicide (Durkheim, 1897/1951).

In the case of Mr. Dancer, the formulation of his plan of action included, along with himself and the case manager, his brother, his daughter, and his physician. With this type of interactive collaboration and assessment, Mr. Dancer had a sense of involvement with the larger community and a greater sense of control over his own destiny that served to build on the earlier buds of empowerment he felt. Through the transaction of drawing up the action plan, Mr. Dancer became aware of the strengths to be found in his formal and informal support systems.

Freud (1917/1955) contended that all depressed individuals have the potential for suicide. In Freud's view, suicide is an intrapsychic process that represents unconscious hostility directed at an introjected, ambivalently viewed love object. To kill oneself is actually murdering hurtful images or memories of one's loved-hated father (mother, friend, etc.) within one's own self (Freud, 1917/1955; Osgood, 1985).

The German word for suicide is *selbstmord* and means self-murder. Menninger (1956, cited in Butler, et al., 1991) believed that the suicide victim wished to die, to kill, and to be killed. In fact, suicide is three times more common than homicide.

Applying the Model to Suicide

According to Freud (1917/1955), the features that distinguished melancholia and profound, painful dejection—for example, the loss of interest in worldly affairs, inability to love, inhibition of activities, and self-condemnation—are ingredients for suicide. Freud's work has influenced other psychological explanations of suicide focusing on the concepts of loss and depression in relation to suicide. In Mr. Dancer's case, the losses he had suffered and his depression were at the center of his assessment and plan of action and individual goals.

To progress toward individualized goals, a practitioner expands the repertoire of resources available to older people. In doing so, the community "is viewed not as toxic but rather as a potential source" of possibilities (Sullivan, 1992, p. 207). For older people this is significant because it encourages their active membership in society while reminding society of their presence.

One of the goals included in Mr. Dancer's personal program plan was to obtain a referral to senior housing, which resulted in a residency that included meals, medical care, and a place where he could have his dog, Tonto, back with him. He was no longer isolated, and began making new friends. Within weeks, he began to spend more time in the kitchen, and got involved with cooking the meals for his fellow residents. This fulfillment of Mr. Dancer's personal program plan demonstrates the innate ability he has to cope, to change, and be self-motivated. Also included as a goal in his action plan was visits to (a) the Social Security office, where he was able to obtain early retirement benefits, (b) the Veteran's Administration office, where he initiated paperwork necessary to secure his pension, and (c) the state Medicaid office, where he obtained eligibility for Medicaid services. Another added touch of community involvement was the use of the local taxi cab that he took to the medical center where he received physical therapy. On one of his visits, Mr. Dancer told the case manager, "Wow, I almost feel human again. I still miss Emma something fierce, but the old juices are starting to flow again and she would like that." An interdependence of relationships was established based on reciprocity, a common purpose, and recognition of the community as a resource. Society rendered resources to Mr. Dancer, and he was able to reciprocate by becoming a full participating member of his community. (See Table 2.1.) This is a good example of how empowerment can lead to membership and regeneration.

The strengths concepts for this case could be mapped as shown in Figure 5.4.

The outcomes of the strengths model of practice are positive for older people and practitioners alike. For older people, the model accents choices, independence, and personal control. The practitioner benefits from having measurable and achievable goals to guide practice (Modrcin, Rapp, & Chamberlain, 1985).

Further, the strengths model, in conjunction with outreach services and crisis intervention, addresses critical factors associated with suicide by stabilizing, engaging, and providing continuous services based on the needs and wants of clients. Mr. Dancer quickly learned that many of his fellow residents had lost their spouses, and he became a member of a bi-weekly grief support group. Here, Mr. Dancer was able to interface with his environment by recognizing the interventions available to him.

Assessment must include determination of suicidal risk. Stress and loneliness as well as other risk factors lead to depression. Table 5.2 provides some examples of risk factors paired to a corresponding strength that can be tapped when applying the strengths model. The risks listed do not carry equal weight and vary according to each individual case.

In Mr. Dancer's case, he experienced nine of the fourteen risk factors listed: bodily changes, loneliness/isolation, helplessness/loss of status,

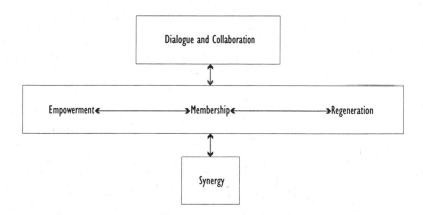

FIGURE 5.4 *Empowerment leads to membership and regeneration*

TABLE 5.2 *Considering Suicide Risks and Strengths of Older Adults*

SUICIDE RISKS	STRENGTHS TO HIGHLIGHT
Bodily changes	History of successful transitions
Alcoholism	History of successful, independent coping
Loneliness	Acquired skills in initiation and forming of relationships; prayer and church affiliation when appropriate
Retirement	Acknowledgment of job endurance/success: opportunity for new life adventure
Helplessness/loss of status	Appreciation of acquired life skills; prayer when appropriate
Decrease in mobility	Cultivate past ability to meet new life challenges
Institutionalization	Acquired ability to share varied experiences, i.e., listening, giving, etc.
Loss of self-esteem	Remembrance of small triumphs
Loss of spouse	Time-tested coping skills
Separation from children	Developed sense of self
Deteriorating health conditions	Recognizes needs from wants; church affiliation when appropriate
Financial stress	Creative management skills
Dependency increase in chronic conditions	Abundance of life experiences; church affiliation when appropriate
Loss of friends and extended family	Reminiscence through pictures; use past skills to make new friends

decrease in mobility, loss of spouse, separation from children, deteriorating health conditions, financial stress, and loss of friends and extended family. The practitioner was able to assist him to see how he could translate most of these risks into strengths. For example, when thinking about the bodily changes he was experiencing, Mr. Dancer was able to recall a time when he had fallen off the roof while attempting to replace some shingles and broken his leg. He had to take a leave of absence from work and let others help him until he got better. He recalled a time of loneliness and isolation when he was laid off from his cooking job of 15 years and was unable to find similar employment. He went to a specialty school, learned how to do French baking, and was able to secure a job at one of the large hotels in town, where he was challenged to form new relationships. When thinking of his present helplessness and loss of status, again he recalled his experiences of strength in dealing with loss of his long-term job. When considering his decrease in mobility, he drew upon his experience of falling off the roof. He had many hours to fill and became an avid crossword puzzle buff. While Mr. Dancer would undoubtedly experience the pain of the loss of his spouse for the rest of his life, he was able to draw on the love and support of his daughter, brother, and fellow residents to help him during his grief.

There are many people in a position to note significant changes in the older adult: children, spouse, neighbor, pastor, rabbi, social worker, nurse, physician. The most logical person, however, is the physician. For example, well over 75% of those older adults who complete suicide have had recent contact with a physician (Clark, 1992; Grollman, 1971; Miller, 1979). Clark (1992) found a high percentage of older adults (over 65 years of age) had physician contact prior to death: 20% within 24 hours, 41% within one week, and 70% within one month, in spite of the fact that the majority were in good physical health. Few of the physicians contacted were mental health practitioners (Clark, 1992).

Depressive conditions are not always easy to recognize. Depression does not necessarily show on a person's face, nor can it be heard in the voice or seen in behavior. Many seemingly normal people carry out their day-to-day lives, smile, express kind words, and remain productive while at the same time struggling with the decision of whether to go on living. Furthermore, older persons experiencing a severe depressive condition have difficulty recognizing their own psychological symptoms because they focus on physical symptoms and physical health concerns. Symptomatic to depression are suicidal thoughts. Persons in acute suicidal crisis often struggle greatly to resist the emotional tug of relieving their pain and of thinking suicide is the solution (Clark, 1992).

Physicians and others in frequent contact with vulnerable older persons must train themselves to look for suicide warnings, diagrammed in Figure 5.2. As Osgood (1985) stressed, "accurate assessment also depends upon carefully listening to and accurately perceiving verbal communications, as well as attitudinal and behavioral changes in the [older] individual...appropriate knowledge of the suicide plan... and lethality potential" (p. 90).

Assessments involving the strengths model do not ignore suicidal risks. However, equal consideration is given to the strengths of older people. For example, chronic or acute depression is recognized as a major factor associated with suicide and is placed in perspective. The senior is given the opportunity to work through the depression step by step, drawing on past successes.

In assessing both risks and strengths, case management is an integral part of the assessment process. The functions of case management in conjunction with suicidal adults are defined in Figure 5.5. In the delivery of the strengths model of practice, case managers are encouraged to join with clients in "naturally occurring community contexts" (Kishardt, 1992, p. 65). This case management approach, often referred to as assertive outreach, shifts the focus from service-centered client programs to client-centered service programs (Rose, 1985). This shift is important for older adults because it serves to empower them, thus helping them to regain control of their lives.

There are numerous positive outcomes from assertive outreach with seniors who are suicidal. First, case managers have the opportunity to gain information concerning the client's environment and to assess the naturally occurring support originating from communities and informal nurturing systems. For example, the practitioner would not have become aware of just how depressing Mr. Dancer's second floor apartment was had she not seen it firsthand. Without the joint family meeting, she would not have witnessed the close ties between Mr. Dancer, his brother, and his daughter.

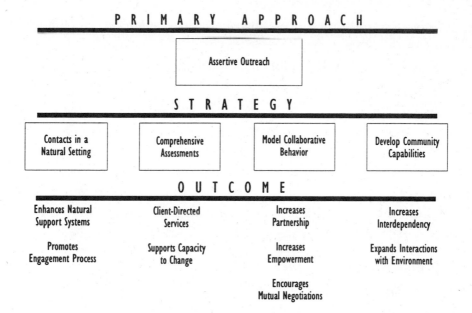

FIGURE 5.5 *Strengths model of practice: Case management with suicidal older adults*

By actually viewing the client's life circumstances, case managers learn of the client's perceptions of life through experience and gather information about the client's life that could not have been known through an office-bound meeting (Mr. Dancer's cooking utensils and pictures of food arrangements). Finally, and perhaps most importantly, the case manager begins to engage the client in unstructured, informal conversations that initiate the helping process in a nonthreatening manner.

If we look at Mr. Dancer and his goodness-of-fit as person-in-environment, we see that the layers of his environment, on initial contact, were in disarray. In his particular time and space, the move into a small apartment from a large family home, his social and physical environment, wheelchair bound and isolated from the treatment community, family, and friends, compounded by his economic circumstance, Mr. Dancer's life was extremely stressful. (See Chapter 2, Figure 2.1.)

After the collaborative assessment, Mr. Dancer began to place demands on the larger society and community for change and support. He did not have to settle for less-than-desirable benefits or conditions. With the collaborative assistance of the social worker, Mr. Dancer pushed on to seek quality of life from his environment.

CASE EXAMPLE

The strengths assessment incorporates two components, process and product. Because of the dynamic nature of these two components, there is ongoing collaborative review and revision of strengths and supports along with conditions. In order to preserve their self-determination, Mr. Dancer and Mrs. M., introduced in Chapter 4, are both subject to the close scrutiny of this assessment process.

Ongoing Collaborative Review and Revision

Mrs. M. slowly began to adjust to her new living arrangement, with plenty of challenges along the way. In early November Mr. M. died. Mrs. M., with the help of her son and daughter, made the arrangements for the funeral and seemed to accept the fact that her husband was gone. After the Christmas holidays, however, Mrs. M. became withdrawn. She reported increasing bouts of insomnia, diminished appetite, and suicidal ideation. "What's the use, Wally is gone for good now and I probably will never get to go back home. I'm a burden on my kids, I don't have a husband to take care of anymore, and I see no reason to live."

Over a 2-week period, Mrs. M. repeatedly said she didn't want to do *anything*, and didn't want outside activities. She said she wanted no day treatment, no outings with her sister-in-law, and seemed to sink more into her depression.

Ms. Morely had to come to grips with her feelings about Mrs. M.'s resistance and apathy about engaging in activities that might ease the depression. She actually began to believe that Mrs. M. was "typical" of many older clients, that is, rigid, set in their ways, and so on, and that Mrs. M. would never change.

In order to further Mrs. M.'s empowerment, Ms. Morely first had to suspend the beliefs she held about older people. Much to her surprise, some negative countertransference issues had surfaced that, if left unchecked, could interfere with continued services to Mrs. M. Ms.

Morely had two aging aunts who suffered from depression and both were obstinate in their refusal of any professional intervention. They called such intervention an invasion of their privacy and held pugnaciously to their views. As a result, one aunt became dependent on alcohol in an attempt to self-medicate and the other spent years in and out of psychiatric hospitals. Ms. Morely was able to achieve suspension of disbelief by returning to therapy for a few sessions and by addressing the residual effects her aunts' behaviors had on her.

Once Ms. Morely gained insight into why her aunts had behaved as they did and why she reacted so strongly, she came to realize that Mrs. M. was not resistant, but rather desperately trying to hold on to the little bit of independence she had left. Indeed, this was a strength of Mrs. M.'s and not a weakness. Again, recognizing and defining clients' strengths and supports is central to collaborative assessment. Behaviors often considered negative, such as resistance, are viewed from a positive perspective; for example, resistance correlates with independence.

Mrs. M. was still new to collaborative interaction, and she told Ms. Morely that she thought Ms. Morely was telling her something was wrong with the way she (Mrs. M.) was coping and furthermore telling her how she should cope with her husband's death. After further dialogue between the two women, Mrs. M. began to see that Ms. Morely was not judging her or dictating her actions, and the stage was set for Mrs. M. to take responsibility for formulating her own goals. There was more work to be done, however, before this could happen. We see again the dynamic nature of the process (Mrs. M. was just beginning to adjust to her new living situation when her husband died) as well as the product: a new life without her husband. This is the new backdrop for Mrs. M.'s life as she and her case manager set about reviewing and revising her strengths and supports.

Through continued dialogue and collaboration, Ms. Morely engaged Mrs. M. in lengthy conversations about her husband and their life together, allowing Mrs. M. to grieve and face some of the cold hard facts about a life without her long-time companion and husband. After many hours and several boxes of tissues, Mrs. M. was able to begin putting some energy toward proceeding with daily living once again.

Ms. Morely encouraged Mrs. M. to discuss her family and social network in a broader context. The ensuing dialogue focused on the accomplishments and potential of Mrs. M., and she was asked to describe specific lifetime accomplishments. In the next three sessions much more of Mrs. M.'s life emerged, including daily life events, financial situations, social supports, physical and mental health conditions, and leisure activities. Mrs. M. began to see more clearly how she handled crises in the past, what she could do well, and whom she felt comfortable with personally and professionally.

Mrs. M. recalled one particular time during the Great Depression when her husband was temporarily out of work and she was able to gain employment in the office of the neighborhood school that her children attended, assisting the nurse and teachers with their daily routines. This sudden recollection gave Mrs. M. a profound sense of empowerment and she gave consideration to the idea of doing volunteer work for one of the local schools. "I really miss my grandchildren; maybe volunteering would do me good."

From this holistic perspective, Mrs. M. was asked to explore what she hoped to accomplish in the next 6 months, divided into 6-week intervals. She decided that she wanted to focus on two life domains at this time, and two individualized personal program plans were formulated. For her first, personal care, she outlined her primary priorities, which included (a) a greater sense of belonging, (b) an increase in purposeful routines, and (c) an improved eating plan. With her wants in mind, Mrs. M. began the process of achieving these wishes through the actions set forth in Figure 5.6.

The first goal in this plan was a different one for Mrs. M. At the time this goal was formulated, Mrs. M. was still experiencing much sadness about the loss of her husband and was ambivalent about her living situation. She still expressed an interest in returning home. "I know it wouldn't be the same without Wally there, and I know the doctor doesn't think it is a good idea for me to be on my own, but I just can't get it in my head that he is gone for good. Sometimes I forget where he is and think he is just late getting off work." Her confusion and short-term memory loss continued to come and go, but she was able to finally

FIGURE 5.6 *Personal Program Plan*

Social Worker/Case Manager's Name
Kate Morley

Client's Name
Mrs. M.

Life Domain:	Living Arrangements	Social Supports	Relationships	x Personal Care
	Education	Leisure/Recreational	Health	Financial

Long-term Goal: Mrs. M. wants to feel a greater sense of belonging. The question that keeps bubbling to the surface for her is "How can I go on without my husband to care for?"

MEASURABLE SHORT-TERM TREATMENT GOALS AND INTERMEDIATE ACTION STEPS	RESPONSIBILITY FOR ACTION PLAN: PROVIDER NAME, LICENSE INITIALS; FREQUENCY; MODALITY; REFERRALS	DATE TO BE ACCOMPLISHED	DATE COMPLETED
Mrs. M. will call the alternative living options that her son and Ms. Morley located and make appointment to visit.	Mrs. M.	March 2	April 16
Mrs. M. will have her grandson take her back to her house to sort through her belongings.	Mrs. M. and grandson	March 2	March 2
Mrs. M. will go to school with daughter-in-law.	Mrs. M. and daughter-in-law.	March 2	April 23
Mrs. M. will plan and prepare one evening meal per week.	Mrs. M.	weekly	ongoing

If more than one page, signatures are required on the last page and are optional on the other pages.

Client's Signature
Mrs. M.
Date   January 26, 1993
Social Worker's Signature
K. Morley, CM
Date   January 26, 1993

Signature and title (other)
D. Moore
Date   January 26, 1993
Signature and title (other)
Dr. Dearheart
Date   January 26, 1993

make the first phone call and make an appointment for her and her son to visit one of the retirement facilities. At that visit she was able to look around and to meet some of the staff and residents. Her ambivalence, however, remained after the visit. "It's okay I guess, but why did that women keep calling the people that lived there 'the dears'?"

Her second goal, going back to her house, was even more difficult. She continued to delay, but finally did go. She spent little time there, but went through some papers and told her grandson to pack up the rest and she'd "deal with it later." The third goal, visiting school, went well for Mrs. M. She said, "I didn't like getting up so early, but I did like being around all the little kiddies." (Mrs. M.'s daughter-in-law worked at a school for teen-age mothers and their babies.) Once again Mrs. M. experienced some confusion, "Now, do my grandkids go to this school?" she asked. After three visits to the school and further dialogue with Ms. Morely, Mrs. M. decided she didn't think she wanted to volunteer there after all. She said, "For some reason it depresses me to be there, maybe later I'll do it."

There was a joint decision, with her son and doctor included, that she would begin to attend the day-treatment program five days a week for awhile. Mrs. M. said, "You know, I think those people over there like me. Maybe we could be friends." Several weeks passed and Mrs. M. announced one evening after dinner, "I don't think I want to move into a place with a bunch of strangers. I have some new friends now and I want to stay here. But you know, I can't quit thinking about moving back to the farm (where she grew up), but I know Dan (her brother) wouldn't have room for me."

Another action step initiated by Mrs. M. was the decision to reactivate her church membership. The church came to be a source of strength and support for her. By taking this step, she renewed her interest in regular Sunday attendance, which expanded into membership in a weekly widow/widower support group.

With this sense of new membership, Mrs. M. was able to continue to deal with the pain of the loss of her husband with the help of peers. Along with the membership she was feeling with her son and his wife, membership in the support group also allowed Mrs. M. to grieve for the loss of dreams originating in her early adulthood. She confided in the group that she had never shared with her family the deep pride she had felt in being able to help them financially during the Depression through her own employment. Nor had she admitted to herself, or to her family, the loss of freedom and security she had felt by giving up that job at the request of her husband after he returned to work. She now wonders whether that loss of brief personal freedom had contributed to the many bouts of depression that followed her throughout her married life.

The preceding assessment is an example of the ongoing collaborative review and revision of strengths and supports along with conditions. Like Mrs. M.'s initial assessment in Chapter 4, it was based on four dimensions: (a) the client's current status (another bottom had fallen out of Mrs. M.'s life with the death of her husband and she felt she had no reason to go on living); (b) stated personal goals (like her earlier goal of wanting to maintain her independence, she wanted to have a greater sense of belonging); (c) internal and external resources (Mrs. M. got in touch with her pain and was able to begin to work through it with the help of others. She also realized the need/want to spend more time with her new friends at the day treatment program); and (d) priority of needs (to "get her house in order" so she could get on with her life, to take steps to improve her eating and sleeping habits, and to continue to work on making her new home a safe, secure place).

Once again, Ms. Morely and the others in Mrs. M.'s life helped Mrs. M. to preserve her right to self-determination. No one forced her to return to her daily activities. She was able to set her own time to return to her house and to call the alternative living facility. This resulted in her making her own decision about remaining where she was and triggered the empowerment she had begun to feel during the summer.

This particular part of the assessment, review and revision, was conducted in Mrs. M.'s home-away-from-home, the day-treatment program in the recreation room. Ms. Morely made tea and served Mrs. M. "I always used to do this for my friends, thank you." While Ms. Morely works in the treatment program and can observe Mrs. M. daily, she changed her role during the review and revision to that of nurturer-friend and served Mrs. M. tea. This temporary role change took her out of her therapist role into the role of friend. This arrangement relaxed Mrs. M., and the dialogue took on a different, more intimate tone, adding to the bank of knowledge of her client.

During those three sessions, Ms. Morely included in her assessment determination of risk regarding Mrs. M.'s suicidal ideation. Using the risks listed in Table 5.2, Ms. Morely helped her client to identify corresponding strengths. They determined that Mrs. M. had experienced five of the fourteen risk factors: loneliness/isolation, helplessness/loss of status, loss of spouse, financial stress, loss of friends and extended family.

Even though Mrs. M. moved in with her son, she experienced great loneliness and isolation from the life she was forced to leave. In response to questions such as, Can you tell me about your best friend? What kinds of things have you always been good at?, and What kinds of things are you good at now?, Mrs. M. talked about her younger sister who had died years earlier and how much she missed her. She recalled that when her sister was living, they would go out together and she made lots of new friends. "It reminds me a little of how I feel about my new friends here." Mrs. M. went on to reminisce about her sister-in-law and how the two of them had stuck together during the drinking days of their husbands. "Maybe I'll give Leona a call." She also talked about how she had left the church because her husband didn't approve, and now she was thinking about going back. As she considered her feelings of helplessness and loss of status, she said, "It's funny not having a husband. The first time I had to tell someone I was a widow I started crying. I know I'm not really helpless, but it sure feels like it sometimes. I remember when I used to go picking berries and make jelly and jam for my family. Maybe I could buy some berries and make jam."

By active listening, reflection, and verbal support, Ms. Morely was able to assist her client to distinguish between needs and wants.

NEEDS	WANTS
1. to grieve loss of husband	to have him back
2. to go home/have a home	a sense of belonging
3. to feel safe and secure	remain with son

NEEDS	WANTS
4. connect with community	go back to her church
5. connect with family	outings with sister-in-law
6. connect with friends	five days at day-treatment program
7. structure in routines	independence

Summary and Evaluation

Once again, through dialogue and collaboration the client was cast in the role of expert in regard to her own unique strengths, interests, and aspirations. Her sense of empowerment began to swell and her membership in the community expanded to include five days at the treatment program, involvement with the church, and grocery shopping in preparation for her weekly meal. As Mrs. M.'s activity level increased, her bouts with insomnia decreased and she began to eat somewhat more.

The process described above allowed Mrs. M. to build on what had worked for her in the past (i.e., church attendance, relationship with sister-in-law, and cooking). The culmination of the review and revision

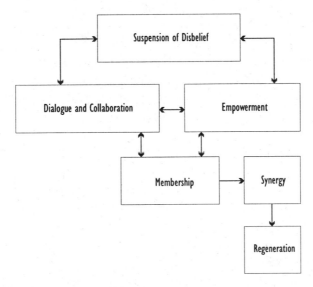

FIGURE 5.7 *Mrs. M.'s process of regeneration*

resulted in regeneration through synergy—the coming together of person and community. Figure 5.7 uses the concepts of the strengths model to map Mrs. M.'s continuing journey.

REFERENCES

Blazer, D. G., Bachar, J. R., & Manton, K. G. (1986). Suicide in late life: Review and commentary. *Journal of American Geriatrics Society, 34,* 519–535.

Butler, R. (1975). *Why survive? Being old in America.* New York: Harper & Row.

Butler, R., Lewis, M., & Sunderland, T. (1991). *Aging and mental health: Positive psychosocial and biomedical approaches* (4th ed.). New York: Merrill Publishing Co.

Canetto, S. S. (1992, Spring). Gender and suicide in the elderly. *Suicide and Life-threatening behavior, 22,* 80–97.

Clark, D. C. (1991). *Elderly suicide.* Final report submitted to the Andrus Foundation, Washington, DC.

Clark, D. C. (1992). "Rational" suicide and people with terminal conditions or disabilities. *Issues in Law and Medicine, 8,* 147–166.

Clark D. C. (1992, April). Narcissistic crises of aging and suicidal despair. *Suicide and Life-Threatening Behavior.* Paper presented as Presidential Address at the 25th Annual Meeting of the American Association of Suicidology, Chicago, IL.

Comfort, A. (1976). *A good age.* New York: Simon and Schuster.

Conwell, Y., Rotenberg, M., & Caine, E. D. (1990). Completed suicide at age 50 and over. *Journal of the American Geriatrics Society, 38,* 640–644.

Cooper, B. (1986). Voices: On becoming old women. In J. Alexander (Ed.), *Women and aging: An anthology by women* (pp. 47–57). Corvallis, OR: Calyx Books.

Durkheim, E. (1897/1951). *Suicide.* New York: Free Press.

Freud, S. (1917/1955). Mourning and melancholia. In J. Strachey (Ed.), *The standard edition of the complete works of Sigmund Freud.* London: Hogarth Press (pp. 237–258).

Grollman, E. (1971). *Suicide: Prevention, intervention, and postvention.* Boston: Beacon Press.

Henery, A., & Short, J. F. (1954). *Suicide and homicide.* Glencoe, IL: Free Press.

Kastenbaum, R., (1992, Spring). Death, suicide and the older adult. *Suicide and Life-Threatening Behavior, 22*(1), 1–14.

Kastenbaum, R., & Aisenberg, R. (1972). *The psychology of death.* New York: Springer Publishing Co.

Kishardt, W. E. (1992). A strengths model of case management: The principles and functions of a helping partnership with persons with persistent mental illness.

In D. Saleebey (Ed.), *The strengths perspective in social work practice* (pp. 59–83). New York: Longman.

Kopell, B. S. (1977). Treating the suicidal patient. *Geriatrics, 32*, 65–67.

Lynn, R. (1969). National rates of economic growth, anxiety, and suicide. *Nature, 222*, 494.

Manton, K. G., Blazer, D. G., & Woodbury, M. A. (1987). Suicide in middle age and later life: Sex and race specific life table and cohort analyses. *Journal of Gerontology, 42*, 219–227.

McIntosh, J. L. (1992). Epidemiology of suicide in the elderly. *Suicide and Life-Threatening Behavior, 22*(1), 15–35.

McIntosh, J. S., & Santos, J. F. (1985–86). Methods of suicide by age: Sex and race differences among the young and old. *International Journal of Aging and Human Development, 22*, 123–139.

Miller, M. (1979). *Suicide after sixty: The final alternative*. New York: Springer Publishing Co.

Modrcin, M., Rapp, C., & Chamberlain, R. (1985). Case management with psychiatrically disabled individuals: Curriculum and training program. Lawrence, KS: University of Kansas, School of Social Welfare.

Morselli, E. (1882/1979). *Suicide*. New York: Appleton.

Osgood, N. J. (1985). *Suicide and the elderly: A practitioner's guide to diagnosis and mental health intervention*. Rockville, MD: Aspen Publishers.

Perkins, K. (1992). Psychosocial implications of women and retirement. *Social Work. 37* (6), 526–532.

Quinney, R. (1965). Suicide, homicide and economic development. *Social Forces, 43*, 401–408.

Richardson, R., Lowenstein, S., Weissberg, M. (1989). Coping with the suicidal elderly: A physician's guide. *Geriatrics, 44*, 43.

Rose, S. (1985). *Advocacy and empowerment: Mental health care in the community*. Boston: Routledge and Kegan Paul.

Sainsbury, P. (1968). Suicide and depression. *British Journal of Psychiatry* (Special Publication), 2, 1–13.

Seiden, R. (1983, November). *Suicide among the young and the elderly*. Paper presented at the annual meeting of the Gerontological Society of America, San Francisco, CA.

Sherman, E. (1991). *Reminiscence and the self in old age*. New York: Springer Publishing Co.

Sullivan, D. (1992). Reclaiming the community: The strengths perspective and deinstitutionalization. *Social Work, 37*, 204–209.

Wolff, K. (1971). The treatment of the depressed and suicidal geriatric patient. *Geriatrics, 26,* 65–69.

Yalom, I. D. (1985). *The theory and practice of group psychotherapy* (3rd ed.). New York: Basic Books.

CHAPTER SIX

Alcohol Use and Misuse in Late Life

THIS CHAPTER IS ABOUT THE EFFECTS of alcohol on older adults and the multiple and varied relationships associated with its use and misuse. Some of the variables discussed include medical complications, early and late onset, use and misuse, acute or chronic alcoholism, addiction, the hidden drinker, and psychosocial implications. The strengths model will be applied, demonstrating assessment and subsequent intervention when working with alcohol related problems.

The Environment, Age, and Alcohol

While estimates vary, there is general consensus that 10 to 18% of older adults in the United States abuse alcohol (Blazer, 1990; Moos, Mortens, & Brennan, 1993). With reference to the 18% estimate, approximately 10% have some kind of drinking problem and approximately 8% are alcohol dependent (Bienenfeld, 1987). Alcoholism is the second most frequent reason for admission of older adults to psychiatric inpatient units (Moos, Mortens, & Brennan 1993). More abused than all other drugs put together, alcohol is clearly identified as the drug of choice for older adults (Blankman, 1993).

Rates of alcohol abuse are higher among younger than older persons, and older men abuse alcohol more often than do older women. However, because alcohol abuse is often hidden among the older population, many incidents of abuse tend to go unreported. The two groups most apt to abuse alcohol are older widowers and men who have never married. Men in veterans' hospitals and domiciliary facilities are, however, also at high risk (Butler, Lewis, & Sunderland, 1991; Maddox, 1988).

ATTITUDES TOWARD DRINKING AND AGING

Evidence of alcohol abuse among older adults is often overlooked. Family members as well as health care professionals are often reluctant to label an older person as an alcoholic for several reasons. Family members and friends may be embarrassed by the older persons' behavior when drinking and attribute the behavior to old age. Likewise, many health care providers are often untrained in gerontology and pharmacokinetics as they relate to older persons and attribute behaviors related to drinking to the natural aging process rather than alcohol abuse (Lawson & Lawson, 1989).

There are certain characteristics of aging that mimic alcohol use, such as memory loss, unsteady gait, confusion, disorientation, and falls (Butler, Lewis, & Sunderland, 1991). In many instances the adverse effects of alcohol resemble some physical diseases or psychiatric and cognitive disorders that are associated with old age. Some examples are complaints of insomnia or restless sleep patterns, irritability, heart palpitations, or a dry cough, all of which can be attributed to alcohol abuse (Hooyman & Kiyak, 1993).

The belief that alcoholism does not occur in older people, held by many health care providers as well as the general public, could also prevent identification (Hooyman & Kiyak, 1993). Another belief held by health care providers and families is that treatment will be unsuccessful in making major changes in the lives of older people: "If you were their age, you would drink too," or "Don't take away their last pleasure" (Blankman, 1993). This line of thinking is ageist. It further denies the fact that older adults are no different from their younger counterparts and deserve the same kinds of treatment.

The case of an older alcoholic client is illustrative. Mr. Wallace, age 73, lives with his 69-year-old wife in their own small, well-kept home. The Wallaces have two children, a son and daughter, who live in the same town. Mr. Wallace was taken to the hospital emergency room for severe respiratory difficulties. The attending nurse noticed that Mr. Wallace had alcohol on his breath. Mr. Wallace was subsequently admitted to the hospital for further observation. The social history revealed the following. Both children were aware of their father's drinking. However, both held differing views about his current drinking practices. Even though Mr. Wallace did not drink as heavily as he had when they were children, the son felt his father still had a severe drinking problem. Because of his father's medical history, chronic heart and respiratory conditions for which his father was taking several prescription drugs, he thought his father should not drink at all. On the other hand, the daughter said, "Gosh, Dad hardly drinks at all compared to the way he used to. He's 73, what can it hurt? I think it gives him one of the few pleasures he has in life right now."

Here is how Mr. Wallace found himself in the hospital ER. He had kneeled down to look at the plumbing under the kitchen sink and was unable to get back up on his own. Mrs. Wallace was able to get him on his feet, but his back "went out" and he had to lie down. His wife tried to persuade him to call the doctor but he refused, saying, "This has happened before and the doctor couldn't do anything. I just have to rest." He began taking pain pills that had been prescribed previously and started feeling better. He quickly used the remaining pills and had his prescription refilled. His wife reported that he was also drinking more than his usual two beers a day. Over the course of one week, despite Mr. Wallace's self-medication, the back pain worsened and he began having trouble breathing. He subsequently had an acute respiratory attack and could not catch his breath.

Mixing alcohol and prescription drugs is not an uncommon practice for older adults. Real health threats are posed when prescription drugs are mixed with alcohol. Because of the potentiating and synergistic effects of combining ethanol with other psychoactive agents, accidental overdoses can occur (National Association of Alcohol and Drug Abuse Counselors, 1993; Vinton, 1991). In Mr. Wallace's case, his self-medication masked respiratory difficulty, which resulted in an acute attack of pulmonary distress.

Characteristics of Alcohol Misuse: Relationship to Environment

Older persons drink for many of the same reasons younger persons do: to cope with physical or emotional pain. As discussed in Chapter 4, old age is the season of losses, and older adults may turn to alcohol, or to more alcohol if already drinking, in order to relieve their pain.

Alcohol abuse/addiction develops in older adults in the same way that it does in the rest of the population in terms of the biological/psychological process of addiction. Actual patterns of use, however, may differ substantially from those of younger adults largely due to the unique psychosocial aspects of aging.

"Alcohol is a central nervous system depressant substitute that adds to impairments that may already exist as a result of various forms of dementia" (Butler, et al., 1991, p. 210). Alcohol indirectly inhibits cortical control, thereby releasing emotional reactions. This inhibition causes impairment of intellectual functions, leading to failure in judgment. At the time Mr. Wallace was admitted to the hospital emergency room, his wife reported that he had taken one and one-half bottles of his prescribed pain medication and one-half bottle of Extra Strength Tylenol®. Alcohol may also affect muscular coordination and bodily equilibrium, which can cause falls and accidents (Butler, et al., 1991).

Alcoholism has been declared a disease by the World Health Organization and the American Medical Association. There remain questions, however, as to the conceptual validity and the therapeutic wisdom of regarding alcoholism solely as a disease. Some believe that a balance should be struck between what is and is not beyond a person's control (Butler, et al., 1991).

There are two distinct lines of thought in the chemical dependency treatment arena. There are those health and mental health professionals who believe in the disease concept and those who do not. The disease concept is seen as a biopsychosocial model and proposes that some individuals are genetically predisposed to alcohol addiction and that this biological vulnerability is exacerbated by psychological and environmental factors (Wallace, 1989; NAADAC, 1993).

On the opposite end of the continuum of the disease concept is the moral weakness concept, meaning that using and abusing alcohol is a sin. Within the continuum there are at least as many explanatory theories as there are definitions of addiction. The three more popularly held theories, psychologic, sociocultural, and biologic, are discussed later in the chapter.

There are other controversies about the nature of alcohol dependency. Some argue that there is no single factor that defines and delineates alcoholism, nor is there a clear dichotomy between alcoholics and nonalcoholics. The sequence in the appearance of adverse symptoms associated with drinking is variable among individuals, with no conclusive evidence supporting the existence of a biological process that predisposes a person toward alcoholism (McNeece & DiNitto, 1994; Pattison, Sobell, & Sobell, 1977). One aspect of alcohol dependency about which there seems to be general agreement is that, whether alcoholism is classified as a disease or not, it dramatically affects the entire family and the subsystems that interact with the family (McNeece & DiNitto, 1994).

SOCIAL, ECONOMIC, AND POLITICAL PERSPECTIVES

There are many social issues related to alcohol use, for example, traffic accidents, other accidents, suicide, the family, and physical consequences (McNeece & DiNitto, 1994; Rivers, 1994). Almost half of the deaths associated with traffic accidents are alcohol related (National Highway Traffic Safety Administration, 1988), as are other accidents such as job-related accidents, aviation accidents, drownings, burns, and falls (Rivers, 1994). Time lost at work, lowered job productivity, health care costs, and treatment related to alcohol abuse and dependence cost our society billions of dollars each year. The projected estimate of these amounts for 1995 is $150 billion (Rivers, 1994; U.S. DHHS, 1990).

There has been a shift over time in the ideology of alcohol use from abstinence to responsible drinking to a public health model (Langton, 1991). According to Langton (1991),

> The current direction of alcohol policy seems to be shifting toward
> restricting the availability of alcohol and toward placing limits on

the advertising of alcoholic beverages. There are at least two new temperance groups which support this policy: the public health advocates who emphasize alcohol and other drug use as a public health problem, and the moralists who emphasize alcohol use as an example for moral evil. (p. 248)

Variables of Alcohol Misuse

Alcoholism for older adults has two categories: early onset and late onset or reactive (Schonfeld, 1993). Early onset individuals are frequently referred to as survivors. They have been drinking most of their lives and have somehow survived the long-term effects. Biological factors are more salient in the etiology of the early onset type: genetic and familial correlations are high. Late onset types typically begin abusing alcohol in later life, often following a loss. In late onset, alcohol is frequently used to self-medicate for such things as depression, loneliness, boredom, and pain (Atkinson, 1990; Butler, Lewis, & Sunderland, 1991; Monk, 1990).

Butler, et al. (1991) offered the following definitions:

> Alcoholism is a condition resulting from excessive ingestion of or idiosyncratic reaction to alcohol. A problem drinker is one who drinks enough to cause problems for him- or herself and society. Acute alcoholism is a state of acute intoxication with temporary and reversible mental and bodily effects. Chronic alcoholism is the fact and consequences of habitual use. (p. 209)

Differences exist, however, between chronic alcoholism and alcohol addiction. The term chronic alcoholism covers all physical and psychological changes resulting from the prolonged used of alcohol, while alcohol addiction is considered a disorder characterized by an urgent craving for alcohol (Bowman & Jellinek, 1942).

The term hidden alcoholic refers to characteristics commonly related to older drinkers. They tend to live in a slower, more isolated environment. Contacts with the community are reduced and negative contacts with law enforcement are rare. As already mentioned, family members and friends tend to be embarrassed by the alcoholic behavior and dismiss it as being related to growing old.

In the case of Mr. Wallace, he does live a much slower life than before retirement, is more isolated from the environment, and has limited contact with the community. He does see his children often, however. At the time of discharge from the hospital, Mrs. Wallace and the children, at her son's urging, discussed seeking outside help to deal with Mr. Wallace's drinking problem. Mother and daughter were ambivalent, but said they would not object. The son made an appointment with the Employee Assistant Program (EAP) provided through his place of employment. His first visit was with the EAP's social worker who, after a brief explanation by the younger Mr. Wallace of the family's situation, asked if the rest of the family would be willing to become involved. They agreed. The social worker, Ms. Hoops, requested that they all meet at the family home to begin an assessment.

At the first meeting the social worker explained briefly the process of the strengths assessment that would be taking place. To help make the family members feel relaxed Ms. Hoops asked each person to say a little bit about themselves and about their view of counseling. Ms. Hoops used a careful and relaxed pace during the session, explaining that during the next few weeks they would be working at the family's pace. She also advised them that she would guide the process but that she was depending on the family to identify the problems and come up with the solutions.

Theoretical Concepts and Environmental Influences

There are vast numbers of theories to explain what causes alcoholism. The more salient ones, however, can be addressed in three broad categories, psychological, sociocultural, and biological.

There are several different psychological theories. Psychodynamic theories offer explanations such as ego deficiencies, with alcohol providing a sense of security. Psychoanalytic theory sees alcoholics as self-destructive, narcissistic, or orally-fixated. Learning theories, also referred to as reinforcement theory, assume that alcohol use results in a decrease in psychological states such as anxiety, stress, and tension, thus negatively reinforcing the user. Personality theories assume that certain personality traits predispose an individual to drug use. For example, an alcoholic personality is often described as dependent, immature, and impulsive (McNeece & DiNitto, 1994).

The basic principle of the biopsychosociological theories is that alcoholics are constitutionally predisposed to develop a dependence on alcohol. Advocates of this theory apply disease terminology and generally place responsibility for the treatment in the hands of medical personnel (McNeece & DiNitto, 1994).

Sociocultural theories, in part, have been generated by observations of differences or similarities among cultural groups or subgroups. These theories tend to attribute differences in drinking practices to environmental factors such as poverty (McNeece & DiNitto, 1994).

TRADITIONAL AND NONTRADITIONAL INTERVENTIONS

Some of the traditional methods of intervention for working with people who have alcohol problems are detoxification, Alcoholics Anonymous (AA), behavior modification, individual, family, or group therapy, and various aversion therapies.

From a nontraditional perspective, it is believed that there is no single superior approach for alcohol problems. Rather, there is value found in a wide range of alternatives, such as education, conditioning, social learning, general systems, public health, and AA. Different types of people respond best to different approaches. There is no advantage to more intensive, longer, or residential approaches over less intensive and less expensive alternatives. Overall effectiveness lies more with alternative approaches and with matching persons to treatment methods, not where treatment is received or how long it takes (Hester & Miller, 1989).

Frequently, in most alcohol treatment centers in the United States, clients are offered a relatively consistent program—the twelve steps of recovery. If clients fail to respond they are blamed for failure because of insufficient motivation. It has been suggested that AA, twelve-step recovery, does not work for certain populations of alcoholics (Hester & Miller, 1989). Kasl's thesis is that AA may not be effective for groups that differ from AA's founders: white, middle-upper-class men. The twelve steps were written for this population with the objective of ego reduction, generally not a necessary goal for people who have been oppressed by racism or sexism (Kasl, 1992).

Applying the Model to Alcohol Misuse

For the nontraditionalists, the question is not which treatments are best, but rather which types of individuals are most appropriate for a given program, or, for a particular individual, which approach is most likely to succeed (Miller, 1992). The emphasis during the initial intervention phase is on motivation and empowerment to help the person to reach the recovery goal. Once that goal has been obtained, the focus shifts to relapse prevention by identifying the person's strengths and resources that are necessary to maintain the recovery goal (Annis & Davis, 1989; Miller, 1992).

According to the National Institute on Alcohol Abuse and Alcoholism (NIAAA), "in contrast to classical, dynamic, insight-oriented psychotherapy, alcoholism counseling is directive, supportive, reality centered, focused on the present, short term, and oriented toward real world behavioral changes" (NIAAA, 1987, in McNeece & DiNitto, 1994, p. 128). The treatment approach defined by the NIAAA lends itself to the strengths model because it addresses people in their environment and aims toward empowerment of individuals.

CASE EXAMPLE

From the family assessment, Ms. Hoops learned that Mr. Wallace had been drinking from the time he was a very young man. During the course of the 2-hour initial assessment, Mr. Wallace became quite defensive several times when his drinking habits were discussed. "Now hold on a minute, I only drink beer and I've told you a hundred times, I can quit any damn time I want." It became apparent to Ms. Hoops that Mrs. Wallace and the two children had talked about Mr. Wallace's drinking frequently over the years, but had rarely confronted him on how his drinking behavior affected the family. "In the early days, the kids and I used to worry when George didn't come home until late, but when I tried to talk to him about it he'd just tell me to mind my business. Eventually I just gave up and started hiding money so I would have enough to pay the rent and buy groceries."

Mr. Wallace had to retire early because of ill health and he said that he didn't drink as much after retiring. The rest of the family, however, disagreed with him, saying that it was only after a life-threatening illness 5 years ago that his drinking slowed down. "I don't know what all this fuss is about," he said, "I've always provided for this family, haven't I?"

After Mr. Wallace retired, he built a workshop behind his house where he did carpentry work for friends and family. It was revealed that he hid his beer in the shop and would sip on it all afternoon. "That's a darn lie," he said, "I only have two beers at the most and not every day. Beside, what's it hurting?"

Mr. and Mrs. Wallace owned their small two-bedroom home. Their only sources of income were Social Security benefits and a modest pension from Mr. Wallace's carpenter's union. The Wallaces had a moderate degree of goodness-of-fit in their environment. Although they lived on a meager retirement income, their home was paid for and in reasonably good condition. Mrs. Wallace was in good health and Mr. Wallace, despite his frail medical condition, continued to enjoy a broad range of activities over the last 10 years up until this recent hospitalization.

The major psychological and social strain experienced by this couple relate primarily to Mr. Wallace's chronic drinking behavior. He was forced to take an early, unplanned retirement because of his ill health 9 years ago. Mrs. Wallace worked part-time as a certified public accountant for 20 years. She qualified for higher benefits from Social Security by making her claim as a wife rather than her own work history. "We don't really suffer financially," Mrs. Wallace said. "We do have to pinch our pennies though and there is not a lot left over after basic living expenses." Mrs. Wallace took pride in her creative grocery shopping. "George and I clip coupons and it really pays off."

Ms. Hoops included four dimensions in assessing the six life domains during the assessment. First, she considered the client's current status. Mr. Wallace was a chronically addicted alcoholic. Mrs. Wallace was feeling frustrated and resentful because of the level of care she provides for her husband. "This has happened before you know. George has been in and out of the hospital many times and the burden of his care always falls on me. I feel like breaking the bottle of beer over his head sometimes." Second, Ms. Hoops took note of the stated personal goals. The initial assessment produced separate goals for this couple. Mrs. Wallace wanted Mr. Wallace to quit drinking and take better care of himself and Mr. Wallace wanted his family to "get off his back" about his drinking. The agreed-upon explicit goal, however, was for Mr. Wallace to recover from his latest health challenge. Third, Ms. Hoops gathered information about internal and external resources. Both Mr. and Mrs. Wallace could be considered as survivors, having lived through many difficulties during their married life together. Their children were both concerned about their parents and very supportive in wanting them to have a good life in their retirement. Mrs. and Mr. Wallace each had several brothers and sisters that lived nearby. Mr. Wallace had a close relationship with his older brother. Last, she assessed her clients' priority of needs. Mr. Wallace needed to regain his health. Mrs. Wallace needed help and support in nursing her husband back to health. With the initial portion of the collaborative assessment concluded, a working relationship had begun.

Descriptive Appraisal

While Mr. Wallace's drinking may have best been explained by reference to psychological theory during his earlier drinking days, it would now appear his drinking was more related to loss and the stresses of aging. Rather than a prescriptive diagnosis, Ms. Hoops provided a descriptive appraisal of Mr. Wallace. It is important to stress again that the prescriptive diagnosis accompanies the clinical diagnosis. Social workers need both in order to provide the client with a holistic plan of intervention. One week after the initial assessment, Ms. Hoops met with the family again at Mr. and Mrs. Wallace's home for ongoing assessment and to institute a treatment plan. The focus was on the family's wants for the future. Before doing this, however, Ms. Hoops gathered additional information regarding Mr. Wallace's drinking history.

From the family, Ms. Hoops learned that all but one of Mr. Wallace's five siblings had a history of alcohol abuse. Two were deceased and one died of complications from her alcoholism, cirrhosis of the liver. Mr. Wallace agreed that he was a heavy drinker and that his whole family is. "It's just our way. When my time comes I'll be ready to go and I don't see what drinking has to do with it." Mrs. Wallace and the children told Mr. Wallace that they believed his drinking had an adverse effect on his health. Hearing this, he became extremely agitated and said, "I'm not going listen to any more of this nonsense." He then stormed out of the room. Feelings were running high and Mrs. Wallace was sobbing, "How can I help him if he won't help himself?"

Ms. Hoops shifted her focus a bit and asked the family members to talk about how they were feeling about what just happened. All expressed feelings of frustration and helplessness about Mr. Wallace's denial of his drinking problem. The daughter and son had some disagreement about how severe their father's drinking really was. According to the daughter, "Once dad calms down I think we can talk some sense into his head." The son said he had tried talking to his father on many occasions and that he refused to admit that he had a problem with drinking. The doctor's report to Mr. Wallace's son indicated that additional drinking on his father's part would have a further toll on his health. After further discussion, they all agreed that they would take a united front and confront Mr. Wallace about his drinking problem.

Ms. Hoops then approached Mr. Wallace in his shop. "I can see that you are upset by what just went on in the house. Why don't you tell me what is going on with you right now?" At first Mr. Wallace refused to speak, busying himself by sanding a piece of wood. After several minutes, Ms. Hoops walked over and asked to see what he was working on. Reluctantly, he turned and handed her the small wooden animal he had been sanding. At Ms. Hoops request, he then gave her a tour of his shop, explaining the various projects he was working on. Ms. Hoops was genuinely awed by her client's fine craftsmanship and told him so. He beamed, "Do you really like it?" he said. "Oh yes, it's lovely, thank you for showing me," she said. She then guided the conversation back to what had taken place in the house earlier. He said, "I know they care about me, but I'm angry and sick to death of them harping at me about my drinking. It's not hurting them one damn bit." "You certainly have a right to your anger," said Ms. Hoops, "and I agree with you, I think your family cares about you very much. Would you be willing to meet with them again to discuss how you might all work together to help get you feeling better?" Hesitantly, he agreed. "Okay, but I'm not going to listen to any more malarkey about my drinking."

The previous illustration is an example of the social worker empowering the client. This was accomplished in two ways. First, Ms. Hoops sought Mr. Wallace out on his own turf and proceeded with the assessment, starting where her client was at the moment. Her approach was gentle but confrontational. Ms. Hoops engaged Mr. Wallace in conversation in his shop, which provided a secure and comfortable environment for sharing personal information. Second, the worker made the client the expert on three fronts: She acknowledged his feelings of pain and anger, recognized him as master of his shop, and put him in charge as to whether or not he wanted to go back to the house and continue the meeting with his family. By empowering the client in this manner, the social worker planted the seed that Mr. Wallace had the resources and capabilities to struggle and survive his drinking and health challenges.

At this point in the collaborative assessment, Ms. Hoops had arrived at a critical juncture. In reviewing what had taken place through her dialogue and collaboration with the Wallace family, she made a list of what had transpired:

- Mr. Wallace is an early onset alcoholic.
- There is a history of alcoholism in Mr. Wallace's family.
- Mr. Wallace adamantly denies his alcoholism.
- Mr. Wallace's health is deteriorating and will continue to do so if he does not stop drinking.
- Mrs. Wallace feels resentful about her husband's unwillingness to help himself.
- The Wallaces live on a modest, but adequate fixed income.
- The couple has many strengths, collectively as well as individually.

As Mr. Wallace sat scowling in the corner chair, Ms. Hoops reviewed the list with the family. Ms. Hoops then received permission from the family to call in Mr. Wallace's physician, Dr. Ball. Mr. Wallace agreed to have a full physical examination. "Absolutely, let him examine me. Then maybe we can put to rest all this poppycock about my drinking effecting my health." When, at a later meeting, the doctor did tell him that indeed his abusive drinking was endangering his health and would undoubtedly shorten his life, Mr. Wallace said, "Bull! You're all ganging up on me and I won't have it!"

Family Plan

Because of Mr. Wallace's resistance to discussing his drinking problem with his family, Ms. Hoops, in a meeting without the client, presented Mrs. Wallace and the children with the possibility of doing a planned intervention on Mr. Wallace; they agreed. Separating the client from the family is atypical of a strengths assessment. In her position as advocate for the entire family, however, the social worker believed the private meeting was for the eventual good of all concerned. Until Mr. Wallace was willing to admit his alcoholism and participate in the formulation of a treatment plan the healing process was stalled.

A planned intervention is a part of the treatment process used by the loved ones of an alcoholic when all else fails. Once the nature of the alcoholism and the magnitude of the denial are understood, the logical outcome is for those caring and responsible people to step in, confront the alcoholic, and propel them into getting help. Intervention is a planned process requiring a trained professional, such as Ms. Hoops, and consists of specific steps. In the first step, each person participating prepares a written list of specific instances in which the loved one's behavior either endangered life, caused embarrassment, or created other problems. The list is specific as to time and place and must accurately describe the drunken behavior and its direct effect on each family member (FitzGerald, 1988; Johnson, 1980).

The meeting was held at young Mr. Wallace's house on Monday morning, as he knew that his dad would be dropping by to help him on a project. This particular morning time was selected because Mr. Wallace usually does not start drinking until midafternoon. Ms. Hoops had briefed the family prior to the meeting, emphasizing that the tone of the meeting must be one of deep concern and that the information must be presented in a totally nonjudgmental fashion.

The intervention was emotionally charged, beginning with Mr. Wallace's rage and incredulity at what was taking place. In the midst of Mr. Wallace's protests, each person presented their list in a loving, caring way, looking Mr. Wallace directly in the eye. He angrily interrupted, frequently at first; however, he remained in the room and his protests began to loose their force once he saw the seriousness of what was taking place and the pain each person had suffered as a result of his drinking behavior. In the end, everyone was crying, including Ms. Hoops. After one hour and thirty minutes of anguish Mr. Wallace said, "Okay, damn you, I'll show you, I'll quit."

The Wallaces' daughter was especially upset and took several minutes before she was able to control her sobbing and speak. She said that she didn't realize the magnitude and extent of her feelings towards her father's drinking. "Hell, I've always said, 'let him drink, he's not hurting anyone,' but making that list really brought out some old stuff. Now I see why I haven't wanted my kids to be around him when he's been drinking. He treats them like he used to treat me when I was their age. He is like a tyrant and a bully ordering me around, acting like I have no feelings of my own. Dad's not the only one that's been in denial."

The next step in the ongoing assessment was for the family to agree on the type of treatment that would be best for all considered. Dr. Ball was included in this phase of the assessment and the meeting took place in a private section of the hospital cafeteria over coffee and donuts. Dr. Ball offered Mr. Wallace much praise and support: "It takes a lot of courage and strength to face something like this, George. I know it is not easy and I'm proud of you. I knew you had it in you." Once again, Mr. Wallace was put in the role of expert of his destiny and further empowered to proceed toward better health. Dr. Ball also told the family that he was convinced Mr. Wallace was depressed and most likely had been for some time. The reason he hadn't mentioned it earlier is because he thought that it was associated with his client's early retirement and that he would get over it. The recent events had caused him to realize that Mr. Wallace had more than one reason to be depressed: His health was deteriorating, his status as a family provider had ended, and since retirement, their monthly income had been reduced by half.

In keeping with the theme of the strengths assessment, the social worker and the clients worked in concert to compile all the salient facts. They worked as a team to identify the client's current status, strengths, and personal goals and wants with regard to each of the life domains. They agreed to regularly update the collected information and to include their perceptions of how things have progressed. The client was placed in the role of expert through nonverbal and verbal communication. Chapter 3 lists seven different ways that this can be accomplished. We will examine a few as they relate to the Wallaces.

Maintain an attitude that is positive and affirmative toward the client. At every opportunity Ms. Hoops and Dr. Ball acknowledged Mr. Wallace's strengths and praised him for his accomplishments, no matter how small. The family received support and positive feedback before and after the intervention.

Conduct meetings in environments familiar to the client such as the home, a park, or local coffee shop. The various segments of the initial and ongoing assessment were conducted in a family member's home or a neutral setting, for example, the hospital cafeteria.

Remain nonjudgmental. Even though Ms. Hoops has been working as an EPA social worker for over three years as a substance abuse counselor, she has had to struggle at times to remain nonjudgmental regarding the process that has taken place with the Wallace family. There is a history of alcoholism on both sides of Ms. Hoops's family and there was an attempt to convince her mother to enter treatment five years ago, including a planned intervention. The intervention in her own family did not proceed as smoothly as Mr. Wallace's, and she found herself judging the various players in the Wallace case throughout the process. Because of her own history, she had arranged with the Wallace family to have a male co-counselor present to participate. She relied on him to help her process the interactions and to provide useful feedback throughout the intervention.

The social worker was able to sidestep some of the difficulties associated with completing a strengths assessment. For example, Ms.

Hoops avoided problem-solving discussions. The worker allowed Mr. Wallace and his family to guide the assessment process. She did not coerce or threaten Mr. Wallace with the consequences of not entering treatment for his alcoholism. Rather she allowed the consequences to become obvious to him through the dialogue and collaboration of the various players, his family and Dr. Ball, regarding his current health status.

As Ms. Hoops explained in her first session with the family, the assessment serves more as a map on a journey toward identifying goals for interventions and seeking the strategies for that intervention together as a team. The social worker then told them of her belief that they were ready, as a team, to proceed with the task of outlining the actual intervention and treatment that would follow.

Studies show that older adults have a higher recovery rate from alcohol treatment than do their younger counterparts (Hoffman, 1989; Mulfork & Fitzgerald, 1992). Just as with their younger counterparts, each person needs to be individually assessed before the proper treatment plan can be decided upon. The treatment plan will vary depending on the multifaceted dynamics of each person and the unique situation. In keeping with the strengths model, alcohol treatment plans establish short-term goals as well as long-term goals. There are inpatient and outpatient services to be considered, with various components in each.

There is ongoing debate concerning the efficacy of age-specific treatment of alcoholism for older adults with two differing views: separate, specialized programs vs. mainstream programs. In a recent study, Schumacher (1993) found little evidence that discrete geriatric alcohol programs were needed for older adults. He does recommend, however, that age-sensitive treatment is indicated and should be accomplished through mainstreaming and the utilization of special tracks for the older adult.

Personal Progam Plan

Even though Mr. Wallace is generally considered an alcoholic, his alcohol ingestion has decreased considerably over the past 7 years and his drinking patterns have changed. He reports that when "all is well" he only drinks two beers in an afternoon. When he is feeling stress, mostly financial, or is depressed, lonely, and down in the dumps, he drinks more. It is apparent that Mr. Wallace has survived the long-term effects of his drinking behavior and is now showing the signs of late onset alcoholism, which results from a series of losses.

The social worker once again placed Mr. Wallace in the role of expert by asking him to select which life domain(s) he wanted to work on first. When he said he didn't know exactly what she meant, she referred to the list she had read to the family prior to the intervention and reviewed it with Mr. Wallace. Ms. Hoops then offered the list to Mr. Wallace and said, "Since your family had the opportunity to make lists about how they felt about you and your drinking, it's your turn to make a list." She asked her client to look at the earlier list and translate it into needs, which he did.

The client then placed the items on his list in order of priority at the social workers request.

1. Have open discussion with his family about his feelings
2. Wants to do more in his shop; use his woodworking skills
3. Will consult with doctor about his health challenges
4. Needs help with his drinking problem

After reviewing his life domains again with Ms. Hoops, Mr. Wallace selected two for his personal program plans: health and social supports. These were the two areas that the whole team agreed were most pressing in terms of actual survival needs in order for Mr. Wallace to regain his health.

As shown in Figure 6.1, the team and Mr. Wallace drew up a personal program plan focusing on the life domain of health. In order for Mr. Wallace to regain his health, he acknowledged that he must quit drinking alcohol. A treatment plan was established, and Mr. Wallace had weekly physical examinations for six weeks, bi-monthly examinations for four weeks, and then monthly examinations. For the majority of the examinations, Mr. Wallace went to Dr. Ball's office, located across the street from the day-treatment program he attended as part of his intervention. The other physical examinations took place at the day-treatment facility.

FIGURE 6.1 *Personal Program Plan*

Social Worker/Case Manager's Name
Maria Hoops

Client's Name
George Wallace

Life Domain: ___ Living Arrangements ___ Social Supports ___ Relationships ___ Personal Care
  ___ Education ___ Leisure/Recreational x Health ___ Financial

Long-term Goal: To stop drinking. To regain health.

MEASURABLE SHORT-TERM TREATMENT GOALS AND INTERMEDIATE ACTION STEPS	RESPONSIBILITY FOR ACTION PLAN: PROVIDER NAME, LICENSE INITIALS; FREQUENCY; MODALITY; REFERRALS	DATE TO BE ACCOMPLISHED	DATE COMPLETED
Work with Ms. Hoops and Dr. Ball to set up a treatment plan to help Mr. Wallace stop drinking	Mr. Wallace, Dr. Ball, and Ms. Hoops	March 22	March 25
Have a weekly physical check-up with Dr. Ball	Dr. Ball and Mr. Wallace	March 29	ongoing
Watch diet; eat less fat and salt	Mr. and Mrs. Wallace	March 22	ongoing
Have some fun	Mr. Wallace and "whoever," "whatever"	March 22	ongoing

If more than one page, signatures are required on the last page and are optional on the other pages.

Client's Signature
G. Wallace
Date   March 19, 1993
Social Worker's Signature
Maria Hoops, BCSW
Date   March 19, 1993

Signature and title (other)
Dennis Wallace
Date   March 19, 1993
Signature and title Dr. Ball
Date   March 19, 1993

Mr. and Mrs. Wallace both began to prepare and eat healthier meals. In the past they had eaten a lot of fast foods and both made a commitment to work at better eating habits for 6 months. Mr. Wallace had a little vegetable garden next to his shop and decided to put in a larger crop that spring. The garden was part of the fun he had stated that he wanted. The other components of his fun were to increase his time spent in the shop doing his crafts and working with his local carpenter's union on their youth project. He also listed watching ball games on television. "Hell, I've always loved to watch a good game, but I don't know how much fun it will be now since I can't drink my brewskies." He did say he would give the games a try though. "Maybe I'll have a bowl of ice cream instead."

In Figure 6.2, the life domain of social supports was the focus of Mr. Wallace's second personal progam plan. Mr. Wallace said he now realized that he had not wanted to talk to his wife or children about feeling stressed and blue because he was ashamed. He thought he could handle it and that it would go away in time. Mrs. Wallace said, "George has never been much of a talker." Mr. Wallace agreed but said he was going to work on it. Mr. Wallace said that he had always wanted to do more of his crafts outside of his shop, but didn't know exactly how to go about it.

The four needs that Mr. Wallace had listed earlier were incorporated into the two plans. All team members participated in drawing up the plans. Note that all family members, Dr. Ball, Ms. Hoops, and Mr. Wallace were part of the team for the domain of social supports and all signed the plan. For the domain of health, only Mr. Wallace, his son, Ms. Hoops, and Dr. Ball were present.

It is critical to capture the details of the client's comments throughout the assessment process. Ms. Hoops did this in several ways. The lists were useful for this purpose. The first one summarized what had transpired in the early stage of the assessment. The first list was later presented to the family, the second set of lists was made by Mr. Wallace's family for the intervention, and the third was the list Mr. Wallace made of his needs. The lists also served to empower the family members by placing them in the role of experts and the social worker in the role of learner in terms of understanding the family as a whole unit.

FIGURE 6.2   *Personal Program Plan*

Social Worker/Case Manager's Name
Maria Hoops

Client's Name
George Wallace

Life Domain:	___ Living Arrangements	x Social Supports	___ Relationships	___ Personal Care
	___ Education	___ Leisure/Recreational	___ Health	___ Financial

Long-term Goal: Mr. Wallace wants to be able to talk more openly with his family, especially when he feels stressed or down. He also wants to have some outside acitvities where he can have fun and can meet people.

MEASURABLE SHORT-TERM TREATMENT GOALS AND INTERMEDIATE ACTION STEPS	RESPONSIBILITY FOR ACTION PLAN: PROVIDER NAME, LICENSE INITIALS; FREQUENCY; MODALITY; REFERRALS	DATE TO BE ACCOMPLISHED	DATE COMPLETED
Mr. and Mrs. Wallace will linger over their evening meal and discuss the events of their day.	Mr. Wallace and Mrs. Wallace	March 22	ongoing
Mr. Wallace will reach out to his children, wife, or Ms. Hoops in times of discouragement or depression.	Mr. and Mrs. Wallace, Patricia, Dennis, and Ms. Hoops	March 22	ongoing
Both Mr. Wallaces will explore outside activities for G. Wallace.	George Wallace and Dennis Wallace	April 23	April 23

If more than one page, signatures are required on the last page and are optional on the other pages.

Client's Signature
  G. Wallace
Date____ March 19, 1993
Social Worker's Signature
  Maria Hoops, BCSW
Date____ March 19, 1993

Signature and title (other)
  Dennis Wallace
Date____ March 19, 1993
Signature and title Dr. Ball
Date____ March 19, 1993

Intervention Plan

The more nontraditional sociopsychological approaches to treating alcoholism in older adults is favored over traditional alcoholism treatment programs because they relate more to the stress of aging. It is also recommended that there be a wide range of community-based programs included in the treatment plan (Blake, 1990). Included in community-based services are informal social support networks, Alcoholics Anonymous, peer groups, and a health component. Clients should be encouraged to participate in social activities, although not necessarily those focused on recovery (McNeece & DiNitto, 1994).

The formal community-based services that became part of Mr. Wallace's intervention were an adult day-treatment program, which he attended on Tuesdays and Thursdays for his depression, and an outpatient alcohol treatment program, which had a special track for older adults. The informal community-based service was Alcoholics Anonymous. Finally, transportation to and from both formal and informal services was considered an additional component. The health component was monitored by Dr. Ball. Mr. Wallace's social activities included working as a mentor-teacher for other union members on their youth project, watching games with his older brother, and regular interactions with his children and grandchildren.

Mr. Wallace's intervention began with a clinical diagnosis, which was done by the treatment team at the alcohol treatment facility. After this was completed, there was a meeting with the key players to discuss the nature of the items that would go into Mr. Wallace's overall treatment plan. Present were Mr. and Mrs. Wallace, Dr. Ball, Ms. Hoops, the team from the alcohol treatment program, the case manager from the day-treatment program, and Mr. Wallace's son. This meeting is an example of how all the various assessments, medical, social, and clinical, fit together to form the holistic component of the strengths model.

As Mr. Wallace progressed in his outpatient treatment at the alcohol center, it was recommended that he attend AA for peer support. He was very resistent to this idea. "I'm not a drunk! Besides, I've heard about those meetings and I don't want to sit around to swap drinking stories. And besides, what if someone recognizes me?" After further discussion about Mr. Wallace attending AA meetings, it was decided that he would investigate whether his union offered any meetings. Mr. Wallace discovered that the union did offer meetings, but after attending three, it became evident that there were no members over the age of 45. Mr. Wallace began asking questions and learned that there were older people who had attended in the past but who didn't return. He was able to obtain a list of older union members who had attended the meetings, called them and stated he wanted to start a meeting for the "over 50." Several expressed interest in this possibility. In the first few weeks only about four or five showed up. By the end of the second month, however, the numbers had grown to eight to twelve attendees.

Mr. Wallace also began participating in his carpenter's union's youth program. When Mr. Wallace and his son were looking for fun projects, they learned that the union had been volunteering their services to the youth at the two battered women's programs in their community. The union's latest project was a fund raiser and they were casting about for ideas. Mr. Wallace suggested that they make and sell miniature wooden animals. He offered his time and his talents to teach interested union members how to make the animals. Mr. Wallace's son offered to help set up an auction at his church to auction them off to the surrounding community.

Mr. Wallace's health domain was also addressed. Dr. Ball had ordered that he wear an oxygen mask for a minimum of three months. At first the treatment was to be daily and eventually decreasing to every other day. This meant he had to make use of a portable oxygen tank and could not drive when doing so. Since Mrs. Wallace was working temporarily for a local tax accountant, she was not available to drive him on the days he wore the mask. The case manager from the day-treatment program arranged to have one of their Retired Seniors Volunteer Program (RSVP) volunteers provide the necessary transportation.

Mr. Wallace's intervention treatment plan contained a nice mix of formal and informal community-based components. In reviewing the components, strengths were enhanced in many ways:

- All formal treatment factions worked together.
- The family, including Mr. Wallace's brother, was involved.

- Mr. Wallace was motivated to organize an AA program to fit his needs.
- Mr. Wallace's talents were used to help local youth.
- Demands were placed on society, for example, transportation.
- Community volunteers were utilized to assist Mr. Wallace.

Summary

The holistic assessment and treatment plan worked well at offering Mr. Wallace and his family services that were not only easily accessed but in which they all played an active part. Active participation reflects the individuality of people and presents opportunities for personal growth, mutual support and an array of relationships.

This holistic orientation has its focus on positive change and out-comes. It supports an empowerment approach to the mental health issues of older individuals by encouraging people to recognize and capitalize on their individual and joint power. Rather than diagnosing and labeling Mr. Wallace an alcoholic or defining his challenges as problems, there was a descriptive appraisal of his needs and wants. Mr. Wallace's assessment and intervention demonstrates how the process is client-driven rather than provider-driven in terms of roles, routines, and rules.

We can see that Mr. Wallace's environment has become a resource for growth and development. Additionally, by shifting the site of serv-ices from an agency location to the social environment his isolation has been minimized. His membership in the community is highlighted and regeneration has taken place.

REFERENCES

Annis, H. M., & Davis, C. S. (1989). Relapse prevention. In R. K. Hester & W. R. Miller (Eds.), *Handbook of Alcoholism Treatment Approaches* (pp.170–182). New York: Pergamon Press.

Atkinson, R. M. (1990). Late versus early onset problem drinking in older men. *Alcoholism Clinical and Experimental Research, 14*, 574–579.

Bienenfeld, D. (1987). Alcoholism in the elderly. *American Family Physician, 36*(2), 163–169.

Blake, R. (July, 1990). Mental health counseling and older problem drinkers. *Journal of Mental Health Counseling, 12*(3), 354–367.

Blankman, B. (1993, January-February). Factors in treating the elderly client. *The Counselor, 11*(1), 17–19.

Blazer, D. G. (1990). Alcohol abuse and dependence. In *Merck manual of geriatrics*. Rathway, NJ: Merck & Co., 1018–1021.

Bowman, K. M., & Jellinik, E. M. (1942). *Alcohol addiction & chronic alcoholism*. New Haven: Yale University Press.

Butler, R. N., Lewis, M. I., & Sunderland, T. (1991). *Aging and mental health: Positive psychosocial and biomedical approaches* (4th ed.). New York: Merrill Publishing Co.

FitzGerald, K. W. (1988). *Alcoholism: The genetic inheritance*. New York: Doubleday.

Hester, R. K., & Miller, W. R. (Eds.). (1989). *Handbook of alcoholism treatment approaches: Effective alternatives*. New York: Pergamon Press.

Hoffman, N. G. (1989). Characteristics of the older patient in chemical dependency treatment. *The Counselor, 7*(2), 11.

Hooyman, N. R., & Kiyak, H. A. (1993). *Social gerontology: A multidisciplinary perspective* (2nd ed.). Boston: Allyn and Bacon.

Johnson, V. E. (1980). *I'll quit tomorrow*. New York: Harper & Row, Publishers.

Kasl, C. D. (1992). *Many roads, one journey: Moving beyond the 12 steps*. New York: HarperPerennial.

Langton, P. A. (1991). *Drug use and the alcohol dilemma*. Boston: Allyn and Bacon.

Lawson, G. W., & Lawson, A. W. (1989). *Alcoholism and substance abuse in special populations*. Rockville, MD: Aspen Publishers, Inc.

Maddox, G. L. (1988). Aging, drinking, and alcohol abuse. *Generations, 12*, 14–16.

McNeece, C. A., & DiNitto, D. M. (1994). *Chemical dependency: A systems approach*. Englewood Cliffs, NJ: Prentice Hall.

Miller, W. R. (1992). *Motivational enhancement therapy manual*. (DHHS Publication, Rockville, MD, Alcohol, Drug Abuse, and Mental Health Administration). Washington, DC: National Institute on Alcohol and Alcoholism.

Monk, A. (Ed.). (1990). *Handbook of gerontological services* (2nd ed.). New York: Columbia University Press.

Moos, R. H., Mortens, M. A., & Brennan, P. L. (1993). Patterns of diagnosis and treatment among late-middle aged and older substance abuse patients. *Journal of Studies of Alcohol, 54* (4), 479–487.

Mulfork, H. A., & Fitzgerald, J. L. (1992). Elderly vs. younger problem drinker treatment and recovery experiences. *British Journal of Addictions, 87*(9), 1281–1290.

National Association of Alcohol and Drug Abuse Counselors [NAADAC]. (1993, February). *NAADAC position statement: Alcohol and the elderly*. NAADAC and NAATP joint legislative conference report, Washington, DC.

National Highway Traffic Safety Administration (1988). *Drunk driving facts*. Washington, DC: Author, National Center for Statistics and Analysis.

Pattison, E. M., Sobell, M. B., & Sobell, L. C. (1977). *Emerging concepts of alcohol dependence*. New York: Springer Publishing Co.

Peele, S. (1989). *Diseasing of America: Addiction treatment out of control*. Lexington, MA: Lexington Books.

Rivers, P. C. (1994). *Alcohol and human behavior: Theory, research and practice*. Englewood Cliffs, NJ: Prentice Hall.

Schonfeld, L. (1993). Research findings on a hidden population. *The Counselor, 11*(1), 20–26.

Schumacher, R. W. (1993). *Certified counselor elderly alcoholism treatment survey*. Unpublished master's thesis, College of Education, University of Arizona, Tucson, AZ.

U.S. Department of Health and Human Services. (1990). *Seventh special report to Congress on alcohol and health* (DHHS Publication No. ADM 90-165). Rockville, MD: Alcohol, Drug Abuse and Mental Health Administration, National Institute on Alcohol and Alcoholism.

Valliant, G. E. (1983). *The natural history of alcoholism: Causes, patterns and paths to recovery*. Cambridge, MA: Harvard University Press.

Vinton, L. (1991). An exploratory study of self-neglectful elderly. *Journal of Gerontological Social Work. 18*(1-2) 55–67.

Wallace, J. (1989). A biopsychosocial model of alcoholism. *Social Casework, 70*(6), 325–332.

CHAPTER SEVEN

Anxiety in Late Life

THIS CHAPTER IS ABOUT ANXIETY AND AGING. By this, we do not refer to anxiety disorder as defined by the DSM-IV-R, but rather a more common form of anxiety that accompanies normal aging. This chapter utilizes the concept of suspension of disbelief and acknowledges that there is a stigma attached to aging—that to grow old in America is to face daily indignation as youth slips from one's grasp. In a society that worships the young, the loss of youth alone can create immense anxiety. Adding the disappearance of youth to all the other losses experienced in late life, there is little doubt that anxiety is attached to aging in varying degrees. The strengths model will be applied to the assessment and intervention of anxiety issues facing older adults.

The Environment, Age, and Anxiety

For many in society, age is seen as a decline or deterioration from youth. The process of aging has come to be seen as a problem to be solved. There is almost an obsession in terms of how to avoid it, for example, through diet, exercise, chemical formulas, or moisturizing creams, and a growing impatience for a final solution to it. Moreover, there are few images of men or women visibly over 65 engaged in any vital or productive adult activity in magazines, on television, or in the movies (Frieden, 1993). It is as though there is a blackout "...of images of people over 65, especially older women, doing, or even selling, anything...in the mass media" (Frieden, 1993. p. 35). The implication is that the image of aging has become so frightening that no one wants to see reminders—reminders that they will never see 45 again and that death may be next. A hopeful scenario is one in which eventually, as more and more people live beyond 65, aging will not be seen as lost youth but rather as a new stage of opportunity and strength (Freiden, 1993). The strengths model of practice lends itself nicely to this anticipated hope and can indeed facilitate it.

SUSPENSION OF BELIEF

> "How old are you?" asks the consulting psychiatrist. The woman tells him that she is 82. "What year were you born?" he continues. "You're trying to check up on me," she says, telling him she was born in 1907. "You're 83," he corrects her. She says, "Young man, I give myself the benefit of the extra year." Next is a memory test, she is given three words—feather, bell and car. Next comes an oral mathematics examination after which he then asks her to tell him the three words. She recalls two. (DeCrow, 1993, p. 11A)

This is an example of ageism and the inability to suspend the belief that all people over a certain age are senile. The psychiatrist stereotyped this 82-year-old woman and assumed she is senile or does not possess all her facilities.

Another example of age stereotyping and not suspending belief is that of an 83-year-old woman who slipped and fell on a wet sidewalk and was taken by ambulance to a hospital, against her will. Her request was to be taken home. She was then told that they must determine why she fell. Young men come and go from her room for several days asking questions. Not questions of Michelangelo, Beethoven, Ibsen, Picasso, or the Democrats, about which she knows a great deal. They ask, "What time is it? (There is no visible clock.) "What day is this?" (There is no visible calendar.) She is not questioned on any topic she has knowledge, information, memory, opinion of, or interest in (DeCrow, 1993).

It is not necessarily the case that some orientation to time and place cannot be helpful when assessing older adults. With a strengths perspective, however, these concerns would not be the focus of a first or even a second visit. What is seen as a priority when doing a strengths intake/assessment is the goodness-of-fit of the person-in-environment. Keeping in mind that the psychiatric assessment has a place in the holistic intervention approach, it needs to be put into perspective within the bigger picture.

The two preceding examples are of women who were not cognitively impaired. Nonetheless, there was an immediate stereotypical assumption that both were senile or otherwise disoriented. Whether an older person is cognitively impaired or not, the above type of questioning and assumption combine to create severe anxiety.

Characteristics of Anxiety: Relationship to Environment

There are many types of anxiety that accompany people into old age. Webster's New Riverside University Dictionary (1988) defined anxiety as "uneasiness and distress about future uncertainties" (p.115). Perhaps a more biopsychosocial definition comes from Tueth (1993), "a diffuse, unpleasant, and often vague feeling of apprehension accompanied by various unpleasant bodily sensations" (p. 51). The term "anxiety" can refer to a mood state, affect, symptom, disorder, or class of disorders (Gurian & Goisman, 1993).

MEDICAL AND PSYCHIATRIC ASPECTS OF ANXIETY

Anxiety in older adults is considered to be similar to anxiety in younger adults, both in etiology and in clinical presentation. Anxiety in older adults, however, is exceedingly complex and while it shares certain characteristics with those found in younger adults, it may be substantially different. These differences are in terms of its presentation and treatment (Salzman, 1991). Primary classifications of anxiety in older adults include situational anxiety, adjustment disorder with anxious mood, generalized anxiety disorder, and phobic anxiety. Another class of anxiety in susceptible patients occurs as a reaction to a number of commonly used prescription and nonprescription drugs. Some of the bodily sensations that accompany anxiety are increased respiratory and pulse rate, sweating, and tremor, along with motor tension exhibited by trembling, muscle tension, and restlessness (Sadavoy, Lazarus, & Jarvik, 1991; Tueth, 1993).

Diagnosing and treating anxiety in the older client is problematic because it does not usually follow a direct stimulus. This means that most older people are generally not aware of their anxiety's source. They are less able, therefore, to reduce it. Anxiety or feelings of apprehension are not always a primary diagnosis. Rather they are more often symptomatic of an underlying mental or physical disorder (Tueth, 1993). While, generally, anxiety complaints are the most common of all psychiatric complaints, both current and lifetime prevalence of anxiety complaints decrease with age for both sexes (Regier, Boyd, & Burke, et al., 1988).

Secondary causes of anxiety, those with organic origin, include medical or psychiatric diseases, drug side effects, and substance abuse or withdrawal (Kendler, Heath, & Martin, 1987). Symptoms of anxiety in older adults frequently are associated with organic conditions and a full medical workup must be included as part of the holistic assessment. Like depression, determining anxiety in older adults is sometimes difficult because they tend to report feelings of physical discomfort when describing their emotional distress.

Anxiety is frequently the primary presentation of almost all psychiatric complaints occurring in older clients. For example, persons with depression, delirium, and early dementia commonly present with anxiety. At the same time, anxiety can mask or hide other psychiatric complaints. It is estimated that 30 to 50% of older depressed clients have anxiety as a major complaint. For instance, in cases such as early stage dementia, clients are usually aware that their intellectual capacities are slipping away, causing them to be distressed and anxious (Cameron, 1985; Sadavoy, et al., 1991).

TRADITIONAL INTERVENTIONS

Once organic causes have been ruled out, the treatment of functional causes of anxiety can be accomplished with psychosocial and/or pharmacologic therapy (Tueth, 1993). In many cases social support, supportive psychotherapy, behavior therapy, and relaxation therapies alone or in combination with pharmacotherapy prove to be effective. Pharmacotherapy, the use of antianxiety drugs, is usually reserved for situations in which anxiety symptoms are severe, of long duration, or fail to improve with psychotherapy (Salzman, 1991; Tueth, 1993). Often, simply changing specific situations can reduce anxiety.

THEORETICAL CONCEPTS

The etiology and pathogenesis of anxiety have been described in various ways. Various schools of thought in this regard include psychoanalysis, behavior therapy, and cognitive therapy. Psychoanalytic theory views anxiety as having a symbolic function that can vary according to its origin; for example, id, separation, castration, or superego anxiety (Nemiah, 1978, and Goisman, 1983, cited in Gurian & Goisman, 1993). Behavior theory views anxiety as an initially classically conditioned response to biological arousal or trauma that is then maintained by avoidance (Goisman, 1983, and Amick-McMullen, Kilpatrick, & Veronen, 1989, cited in Gurian & Goisman, 1993). Cognitive theory views anxiety-producing thoughts, no matter the origin, as both expressing preexisting anxiety and in themselves causing or increasing anxiety (Beck & Emery, 1985, and Barlow, 1992, cited in Gurian & Goismen, 1993).

While fully recognizing the importance of screening for organic causes of anxiety and the existence of chronic, preexisting anxiety complaints, this chapter places its focus on situational anxiety. "Situational anxiety is an exaggerated reaction to common life experiences" (Tueth, 1993, p. 52). Some typical examples of the differing types of situational stressors that might facilitate an anxiety reaction in an older person are: (a) financial—will there be enough money to live on? Where is the money coming from? (b) physical—declining vigor; diminished sensory and functional capacities. Will there be unexpected illnesses? If so, will the person be able to care for him/herself? and (c) loss and loneliness—increasing dependency and fear of isolation; Will there be family and friends for companionship? More subtle examples of situational anxiety can be found in such things as waiting: for a ride, someone to provide assistance, a phone call to be returned, someone to return home, dinnertime, bedtime.

Applying the Model to Anxiety

As with depression, the strengths perspective views situational anxiety as an unexpected reaction to life conditions that occurs in older and younger adults alike. For example, a 35-year-old divorced woman could be equally as anxious as a 74-year-old widow about paying the rent and buying food if her monthly check was late coming.

CASE EXAMPLE

Mr. and Mrs. Truman lived in a medium-sized community in the small, two-bedroom home they have owned for 50 years. Mr. Truman was 79, Mrs. Truman 74. They had one daughter who lived in a nearby town 65 miles north of their home. Both the Trumans were in reasonably good health until the past few years. Mr. Truman suffered a congenital heart attack last year. He recovered, however, and experienced limited vitality as a result. Mrs. Truman began having problems related to her heart about 6 months before assessment, which drained her of her physical and emotional stamina. The severity of her heart condition is such that surgery is not considered useful in correcting the problem. The doctors told the family that Mrs. Truman's condition will be stable for approximately 1 to 3 years. Subsequently, it was not expected that she would be capable of caring for herself, even with the help of her husband. The daughter, Mrs. H., requested the services of a home health agency to assist the family in making decisions about short- and long-term care for her mother.

A social worker, Ms. Kelly, and a nurse practitioner, Mr. David, were assigned to the case. Ms. Kelly completed the strengths assessment and Mr. David completed the medical assessment. Both Ms. Kelly and Mr. David were present for the strengths assessment, which was done in the Truman's home. Also present were Mrs. Truman's daughter and son-in-law, Mrs. and Mr. H. It was learned that Mrs. Truman had recently expressed a desire to move to the town where her daughter lived. She believed that it was far too burdensome for her daughter to continue the long commute to care for her and Mr. Truman at each misfortune they experienced. Mr. Truman, however, had never been keen on relocating. "This house represents everything in my life for the last 50 years. I'll be damned if I'm going to sell it and move into some dinky apartment. Mother and I can manage by ourselves. The neighbors have been pretty darn good about lending us a hand."

The debate about moving continued for several weeks and tempers flared more than once. "If the Lord is going to call me home soon, I want to enjoy what time I have left and I want that time to be with my daughter and grandkids close by," said Mrs. Truman. Mr. and Mrs. H. also wanted the Trumans to move. They were both employed and Mrs. H. had used almost all of her leave time during the previous six months traveling to care for her mother. "My wife is tired all the time what with working and trying to manage her own life," said Mr. H.

Ultimately, the family decided, albeit reluctantly on Mr. Truman's part, that the Trumans would move north. They put their house up for sale. Mrs. and Mr. H. located a condominium near their own home for the Trumans and borrowed money to place a down payment on it. Throughout this process, both Mr. and Mrs. Truman experienced a great deal of anxiety. Mrs. Truman had an increased pulse rate, had trouble eating, was restless, and didn't sleep. Mrs. Truman said, "All Hank does is pace back and forth between the kitchen and the living room, back and forth, back and forth. He's driving me crazy with the pacing. And, beside that, he is grouchy as an old sow." Mr. Truman replied, "Nag, nag, nag, that's all she ever does, picks at me on every-thing little thing I do. Nothing ever seems to please her."

During one of the visits from the home health team, Mrs. Truman commented that she was "nervous as a cat" and was fearful that she was loosing her mind. Mr. David reviewed her medical assessment again and reevaluated her medication regimen. He discovered that two of her medications, one prescription, one nonprescription, had properties that could add to her anxiety. He conferred with her physician, who agreed to evaluate Mrs. Truman's medications.

It was learned that Mrs. Truman's doctor had prescribed Valium for her. Her daughter was very concerned about this, saying, "I know Mom is nervous, always has been, but this drug is not working for her. Either she is a zombie or high as a kite. I think she is depressed." Mr. David conveyed this to the doctor, and during a later visit he discontinued the Valium and prescribed an antidepressant with somewhat better effect.

The time arrived for Mr. and Mrs. Truman to go north and look at the condominium. On the trip north, Mrs. Truman was happy, almost giddy, and Mr. Truman was withdrawn and sullen. On the return trip, after looking at the condo, both were quiet. The next day Mrs. H. received a call from her mother, who said, in a very calm voice, "We are not going to move, I can't live in a house that pink. I know you are disappointed, and that you spent a lot of time helping us out in this matter, but we can't do it. Forgive me, goodbye." Mrs. H. called Ms. Kelly, very upset and in tears. "What in the hell do I do now? I'm furious with my mother. My husband and I have put a down payment on this condo, I'm exhausted and cannot keep going back and forth. I'm at my wits end. If they won't move I just don't see how I can continue to help them." Ms. Kelly suggested a family meeting. This meeting again took place in the Trumans' home with Ms. Kelly, Mr. David, the Trumans, and the Hs.

After a tearful, emotional hour-and-a-half session, it was revealed that Mrs. Truman had only agreed to move to please her daughter. She said, "It just kills me to see Barbee so tired all the time, and I know that with me getting sicker every day she will only have more traveling to do. I thought it would be the right thing to do, but after I saw the place, all those pink walls, the tiny little yard with the high fence around it, lordy, my heart just sunk." Mr. Truman was crying. Through tears, he said, "I never liked the idea but decided to go along with it because I don't know what to do anymore. I just wanted Mamma to be happy. I feel so tired these days and my mind doesn't seem to work like it use to. I just can't think through things like before."

Through dialogue and collaboration, Ms. Kelly helped the family see that it is not really the pink walls or the condo itself that created all the Trumans' anxiety, but rather the act of releasing the last bit of independence that remained to them. Being unable to live inde- pendently in their own home would strip them of a tremendous sense of self-identity and security which they felt in their own little corner of the world—their house and neighborhood. The reality of moving north and leaving their life behind them shook the foundation of that security, causing their anxiety and subsequent reactions. Mrs. H. came to realize that wanting her parents to move wasn't sufficient reason for them to do so. Her parents had to want to move also. In spite of her anger and resentment, Mrs. H. was able to see the logic in what had happened. After a few more sessions, Mrs. H. was able to work through her fury and disappointment, and Mrs. Truman was able to forgive herself for disappointing her daughter. "It's eating me up inside, the guilt I feel about letting Barbee down. It's really killing me," said Mrs. Truman.

It was evident to Ms. Kelly that Mrs. H. and her mother had a very close bond with one another and that both felt guilty for not being able to make the other happy. Mrs. H. felt an especially heavy responsibility because she was the only one to care for her parents and she worried that she would not be able to continue to know what was best for them. Ms. Kelly learned that this family had a strong belief in God and encouraged them to pray together, which they did. Both Mrs. H. and her mother said that the prayers gave them comfort and a new sense of direction.

Spiritual or religious assessment has a meaningful place in the strengths model. It is part of the holistic picture that the model adheres to: strength, hope, and a belief in self. The strengths model views the client as being in an environment that provides a holistic approach to community resources. Likewise, social workers assist clients in tapping all the inner resources available to them as whole persons. It has been only in the last decade that social workers and other mental health professionals have begun to realize the importance of including the spiritual or religious dimension as part of the whole person—physical, mental, emotional, *and* spiritual (Canda, 1988; Cowley, 1993; Serma-beikian, 1994).

By including Mrs. Truman's religious beliefs and feelings as part of the collaborative assessment, Ms. Kelly provided her client and her client's daughter, Mrs. H., with a way to tap into their inner resources for help and guidance. Both were feeling frustrated and helpless in trying to solve the problem caused by the miles that seemed to be causing a barrier to their immediate relationship. The intimacy of their prayers together softened that barrier by reaffirming their love for each other and the faith in their ability to generate a solution to their problems.

In a subsequent telephone conversation with Mrs. H., Ms. Kelly learned that she had spent many sleepless nights agonizing over what to do about her parents. She said, "Mom, who I am having such difficulty letting get old and sick, is having great difficulties herself. The test results did shake me up, however. God has given me a calm, peaceful sense. I pray each moment for guidance. It seems that 'the Plan' should include 'it will get easier as you age' not 'it will get harder.' This is not just an experience in caring for a sick parent, it is a time filled with emotions of watching my parents—my strong, guiding, ever-present parents—and realizing they are frail, dependent, old persons who now need my guidance. Nonetheless, I can't help but feel angry and be-trayed, while at the same time knowing Mom feels exposed and threat-ened. Gosh, I feel so confused, so conflicted."

The case managers could see that Mrs. H. was reaching the limit of her ability to continue as the sole caregiver for her parents. Ms. Kelly and Mr. David chose, at this juncture, to offer as much assistance and guidance to Mrs. H. as possible while they explored other informal support systems. At the beginning of assessing informal supports, it appeared that Mrs. H. was the sole support. After a brainstorming session, however, the resources broadened considerably.

The strengths model considers the client's well-being as being largely determined by their resources of informal supports, including those in the community. These informal systems are recognized as being untapped resources with abundant potential for clients and typi-cally consist of unpaid family members, friends, and community op-tions. In other words, older persons' strengths are matched with normal and naturally occurring resources such as family, friends, youth groups, and Rotary clubs before paid services are used (Modrcin, Rapp, & Chamberlain, 1985).

As discussed in Chapter 2, identifying these informal resources is accomplished by including the following questions in the assessment:

(a) Who comprises the client's family members and friends and how capable are they to meet the client's needs and wants? (b) in what ways do the components of the informal system interact with one another and with the client? (c) in what ways does the informal system support the client? and (d) what are the client's community affiliations?

Although Mrs. H. was an only child, she had three adult children who were devoted to their grandparents. Two of them lived in the same town as Mrs. H. The Truman's nephew also lived in their community and was very concerned and available to assist them when he could. The Trumans' next door neighbors had lived in the neighborhood as long as the Trumans. Although they were also aging, they remained a great source of help and support for the Trumans. All of these informal systems had a high level of interaction with the Trumans and expressed their willingness to help out in whatever ways they could. The clients' community affiliations, however, were found to be minimal at the time of the assessment.

Because the Trumans were not moving, Mrs. H. needed assistance in caring for her parents. It also became evident that the Trumans were not aware of what resources were available to them. The social worker, Ms. Kelly, took on the role of educator and advocate while reinforcing the Trumans in the decision-making process.

Ms. Kelly and Mr. David, along with the Trumans, the Hs and their oldest daughter, Rexena, began brainstorming for resources. They approached this task in a somewhat systematic way by first listing all family members they thought might be available. They then considered friends, neighbors, professional associates, and then other significant individuals as sources of support.

Part of the advocacy role in developing resources involves influencing resource persons and networks to be more responsive to the unmet needs of older clients. Such networks might include social services, medical, legal, and mental health systems (Kisthardt 1992). Lustbader and Hooyman (1994) have provided a list of potential helpers and include nurses and receptionists at doctors' offices, bus drivers, apartment managers, grocery store clerks, postal carriers, delivery persons (fuel, meals, groceries), pharmacists, restaurant staff, and others.

The team's resulting list included more informal resources than the Trumans had ever imagined existed for them. In addition to supporting the Trumans as they moved toward setting the goals necessary to enable them to remain at home in their community, Ms. Kelly provided just enough assistance to allow them to remain in the expert position.

Ultimately, the Trumans' informal support system appeared as follows:

1. **Family** Mrs. and Mr. H., two of their children, Rexena and Marcus, the Trumans' nephew, Paul, and, Mr. Truman's sister-in-law, Janess.

2. **Friends and next-door neighbors** The Careys.

3. **Professional associates** Both the Trumans had been seeing the same family doctor for 20 years and they had become favorites of the support staff. The staff agreed to help with the completion of insurance forms and with arranging for transportation when needed. The drug store where they shopped offered extended terms for bill payment and their pharmacist agreed to ensure that they both understand the directions for taking their medications as well as instructing them on possible side effects. The drug store manager indicated that it would be possible to deliver the Trumans' medication on Wednesdays.

4. **Others** The grocery store, postal carrier, meter reader, and restaurant staff. The grocery store clerks agreed to assist the Trumans in their shopping and to cash their social security checks for them. The postal carrier said that he would ring the bell and hand-deliver the mail. In this way, he would be alerted to any possible difficulties in the house. The woman who read their gas meter said that she would inform them when she would be coming and would deliver certain items they might need at that time. She stated that she would also do some "friendly visiting" for 15 to 20 minutes at each visit. The staff at the McDonalds, where the Trumans always had breakfast, said that they would assist in any special food preparations that the Trumans might require, would offer them discounts, and would extend credit for an additional month if necessary.

Through the team approach of the social worker and the nurse, as well as the other auxiliary formal supports, this family's short-term goals were met and the long-term goals were established. The strengths assessment, through engagement, continuous collaboration, and support, generated a holistic profile of the Trumans and their family. The focus of the intervention was placed on the Trumans' strengths, not their problems. The following is a comparison of problems and strengths, demonstrating that the strengths were pursued by Ms. Kelly and Mr. David.

PROBLEMS	STRENGTHS
1. Mrs. Truman's failing health.	1. Health failing, but still very much okay with life.
2. Informal support system 65 miles north, daughter less and less able to continue to help.	2. Daughter 65 miles away, but very devoted and committed to making the situation work.
3. Mrs. Truman wanting to move (so she thought).	3. & 4. Mr. and Mrs. T. willing to explore alternatives even though both are not in agreement of desired outcome.
4. Mr. Truman not wanting to move.	
5. Both reneged on move.	5. Family pulling together to remedy the situation.
6. Emotional pain and guilt for not meeting others' needs.	6. Faith in God and prayer to help them through.

Through this comparison of problems and strengths, the wants of the family members are also highlighted. Mr. and Mrs. Truman's wants were:

1. to make their daughter happy

2. to be safe and secure

3. to carry on with their lives as they have done for the past 20 years to the best of their abilities for as long as they can

Mrs. H.'s wants were:

1. for parents to move north

2. for parents to be safe and secure

3. for her and her parents lives to be less hectic

Ms. Kelly further pursued with the family past strengths of the Trumans that helped them along their life's journey. For example, when Mr. Truman had a sick spell that caused him to be out of work for over a year, Mrs. Truman worked temporarily to maintain the family income. This temporary position led to further part-time employment, which not only helped out financially, but provided her with a deep sense of fulfillment.

Another strength that surfaced was Mrs. Truman's love of sewing. "My, yes, I made all of Barbee's clothes when she lived at home. Then I made them for the grandkiddies. Don't have the patience for it anymore, though." It was revealed that Mr. Truman was very much the handyman and had worked on things around the house and yard, as well as on the car. Although both the Trumans have lost interest in doing these types of activities, Ms. Kelly pointed out what gifts those skills are and how much satisfaction each had derived from doing them. Through further dialogue and collaboration, Ms. Kelly helped them tailor these foregone talents into current satisfying activities.

Mrs. Truman decided to engage again in the hobbies she formerly enjoyed utilizing her sewing talents. Mr. Truman made a list of things that he believed he could do around the house. This was a two-part list. He could perform half the list alone while half required assistance. Rexena said that she would be thrilled to help her Grandpa out.

Individual achievements and skills that were once consumed in the process of survival are now being translated into strengths that can be adapted into tools that will enrich the Trumans' life as they continue their journey into old age. Personal growth will continue for both of them, providing them with ways to reduce the anxiety that will undoubtedly accompany them.

Throughout this collaborative exploration of these talents, Ms. Kelly put the Trumans in the role of experts in each of their life situations. With this emphasis on strengths and resources, the problems were put into perspective and the pressing question shifted from the kind of life they once had to what kind of life they wanted now. This type of approach also suspends the belief that older people are not capable of solving their own problems when they have the support and understanding of others who care.

Earlier, the family members were also put into the roles of experts. After the Trumans decided that they wouldn't move north, Ms. Kelly collaborated with the entire family on alternatives, helping them to reframe the problem into action plans.

Summary

The life domains focused on were health, living, and social supports. The short-term goals were to educate the family and the Trumans regarding the specifics of Mrs. Truman's heart condition, to establish ways in which the family could work together to provide mutual support for Mrs. Truman as her heart condition progressed, and to brainstorm on the roles of the various players. The long-term goal was to put informal and formal resources into place to enable the Trumans to remain in their home for as long as possible.

One week later, Ms. Kelly received a thank-you card from Mrs. H. with the following poem she had written about her parents and a note:

> I have observed the
> bitterness/love
> completion
> despair/sadness
> uncertainly/certainty
> quilt,
> pathetic-frail
> aggressive-frail
> nature of each
> and between each

> Thank you so much for your assistance in helping with Mother. I'm not sure how we would have made it through these difficult times on our own. I felt like you always respected what we had to say. It was truly refreshing to be asked what we wanted, where we wanted

to be in terms of services at various times, and what we wanted to do. We didn't feel forced into doing things and it was reassuring not be rushed. I am especially appreciative of that long talk you and I had the day you walked me out to my car after Mom had decided she didn't want to move. I was about as low as I've been through this entire process and having you share with me about what happened to you and your mother meant a lot. At times I thought I was the only one who has ever experienced something this painful. I now know differently.

REFERENCES

Cameron, O. G. (1985). The differential diagnosis of anxiety: Psychiatric and mental disorders. *Psychiatric Clinical North America, 8*, 8–20.

Canda, E. (1988). Spirituality, religious diversity, and social work practice. *Social Casework, 69*(4), 238–247.

Cowley, A. S. (1993). Transpersonal social work: A theory for the 1990's. *Social Work, 38*(5), 527–535.

DeCrow, K. (1993, November 23). Harassing the elderly. *USA Today*, p. A11.

Frieden, B. (1993). *The fountain of age*. New York: Simon & Schuster.

Gurian, B., & Goisman, R. (1993). Anxiety disorders in the elderly. *Generations, 17*(1), 39–42.

Kendler, K., Heath, A., & Martin, W. (1987). Symptoms of anxiety and symptoms of depression: Same genes, different environment? *Archives of General Psychiatry, 44*, 451–457.

Kisthardt, W. E. (1992). A strengths model of case management: The principles and functions of a helping partnership with persons with persistent mental illness. In D. Saleebey (Ed.), *The strengths perspective in social work practice* (pp. 59–83). New York: Longman.

Lustbader, W., & Hooyman, N. R. (1994). *Taking care of aging family members*. New York: The Free Press.

Modrcin, M., Rapp, C., & Chamberlain, R. (1985). *Case management with psychiatrically disabled individuals: Curriculum and training program*. Lawrence, KS: University of Kansas, School of Social Welfare.

Regier, D. A., Boyd, J. H., Burke, J. D., et al. (1988). One-month prevalence of mental disorders in the United States. *Archives of General Psychiatry, 45*, 977–986.

Sadavoy, J., Lazarus, I., Jarvik, L. (1991). *Comprehensive review of geriatric psychiatry*. Washington, DC: American Psychiatric Press, Inc.

Salzman, C. (1991). Conclusion. In C. Salzman & B. D. Lebowitz (Eds.), *Anxiety in the elderly: Treatment and research* (pp. 305–312). New York: Springer Publishing Company.

Sermabeikian, P. (1994). Our clients, ourselves: The spiritual perspective and social work practice. *Social Work, 39*(2), 178–183.

Tueth, M. J. (1993). Anxiety in the older patient: differential diagnosis and treatment. *Geriatrics, 48*, 51–54.

Webster's New Riverside University Dictionary. (1988). [2nd ed.]. Boston, MA: The Riverside Publishing Co.

CHAPTER EIGHT

Work, Retirement, and Leisure from a Strengths Perspective

A FREQUENTLY ASKED QUESTION ABOUT the strengths model is: Who uses it and in what settings/agencies does it apply? The answer is both simple and complex. It is simple in that anyone working with people can use a strengths perspective. In fact, many mental health providers are already using some of the concepts contained within the model. The answer is complex in terms of the setting or agency. The complexity is not in the use itself, but rather in how to insert strengths into the already existing medical model with its focus on problems and weaknesses. Chapters 4 through 7 discuss the application of the model in a variety of settings and agencies with a variety of practitioners using a micro approach to intervention. Chapters 8 and 9 turn to more of a mezzo and macro approach of intervention and prevention.

As the number of retired individuals in the population increases, the need to recognize their unique talents and skills also increases. As people live longer lives, many will spend as much time in retirement as they did in the workplace. Since retirement is almost exclusively the domain of older adults, it is a necessary topic for discussion in this book. In this chapter, framed within the strengths model, the perspective of prevention is used to examine the concepts of work, retirement, and leisure as a process rather than as singular events. Prevention is seen here as a tool for reducing stress, anxiety and depression, and enhancing the mental health of older adults.

Many of the terms discussed in this chapter beg for definition, that is, old age, work, retirement, prevention, leisure, religion/spirituality, and quality of life/life satisfaction. There are also many questions that arise. For example, what constitutes old age, is work paid or unpaid, when does retirement occur and what form does it take, what does leisure consist of, and what constitutes quality of life? Further discussion may yield some answers.

What is old age, how old is old, and who defines it? Ironically, as controversial as growing old and "old age" is, it is arbitrarily defined by policy. Social legislation of the 1930s decreed 65 as the age when one would retire and become eligible for various services available to older persons. While retirement legislation has changed, abolishing mandatory retirement, age 65 has stuck as the age of "obsolescence."

Building on the notion from Chapter 7 that aging is a natural process and not something that must be cured, the strengths model places more emphasis on the fact that growing old *does not* mean obsolescence, an end. Rather than blindly focusing on the beginning and the middle, more attention must be paid to the concept of life span development which does have a beginning, middle, *and an end*. When aging is denied as a natural part of the sequence of the life span, it is not only older persons who suffer. Erikson (1963, quoted in Daniel, 1994, p. 62) states that "[L]acking a culturally viable ideal of old age, our civilization does not really harbor a concept of the whole of life." Young people need models to show them how to plan for their whole lives, how to gain insight into themselves, and how to develop spiritually (Daniel, 1994).

Work

What is work? Examples include paid work—employment—and unpaid work. Unpaid work takes many forms: homemaking, parenting, caretaking of old or sick friends and relatives, volunteering time, and some hobbies and avocations. Both will be discussed. We turn to discussion of paid work first. In fact, any discussion of retirement must be placed in the broader context of lifelong work experience.

Work force participation is an economic predictor for retirement. This prediction is especially significant for working-class men and women who have experienced labor market inequities (Atchley, 1982a; Perkins, 1993a). For women, evidence of this inequity is found in the fact that 77% of all employed females are working in low-pay occupations and industries (National Commission on Working Women, 1986). This trend is expected to extend into the next century. As will be seen in Chapter 10, however, the trend will be somewhat different for the nation's baby boomers as they move toward retirement age. Nonetheless, this currently leaves scores of older women retiring into poverty (Perkins, 1993b). Women are especially hard hit, not only because they outlive men, but also because they often outlive their assets.

When women are examined within the broader context of lifelong work patterns, a clearer picture of their economic status emerges. Women frequently have interrupted work histories, specifically for reasons of caring for family members, and hold either part-time or low-paying, low status jobs (Perkins, 1993b). The poorest category among all the older adult groups is African American women (Gould, 1989).

Social Security and pension systems will have practically ended poverty among older men and couples by the year 2020. Poverty will remain widespread, however, among older women living alone, divorced, widowed, or never married (Older Women's League, 1990). Poverty income guidelines in 1992 revealed that for a family of one, income less than or equal to $6,729, and for two, less than or equal to $8,487 signified an existence at or below poverty existence (U.S. Bureau of the Census, 1992).

The Social Security Act, drafted more than 50 years ago, best protects a family consisting of a lifetime paid worker, typically a husband, a lifelong unpaid homemaker, typically a wife, and dependent children. Seventy percent of older, nonmarried women, however, depend on Social Security as their sole income. This system is obviously outdated, and if left as it stands, future generations of women will continue to receive Social Security benefits that are significantly inadequate (Older Women's League, 1990).

The work lives of men and women are increasingly similar. Both seek feelings of competence, of making a contribution, of being necessary and productive, and of being in control of time and energy. The differences, however, are significant with regard to earnings and occupations (England & Farkas, 1986; Perkins, 1992). Women and men are the same in that earnings are crucial to personal support and to support families (Levitan, Mangum, & Marshall, 1976; Report on Status of Midlife and Older Women, 1986). Women and men are not the same, however, in the amount of earnings they receive.

Women's salaries are not commensurate with those of men. Rather, women's earnings are substantially less (Older Women's League, 1986). Women have earned an average of $0.64 for every $1.00 earned by men consistently since 1950 (Smith & Ward, 1984; Faludi, 1991). This gap has closed slightly (about 10%) in the past decade, due not to salary increases for women but to the decline in men's salaries (Cory, 1993).

Not only are there economic differences related to gender in the work force, there are differences related to race. African American women have a narrower sex-wage differential than white women due to the interaction of race and sex discrimination in hiring and promotion (Madden, 1985). Bergmann (1971) suggested that race discrimination can cause wage differentials among equally skilled occupations and that wage differentials by race may be maintained through occupational segregation rather than overt wage discrimination.

An examination of differences in work histories among male and female African American and white adult workers found African American women's work histories to be less continuous than those of African American and white males. African American women's work histories were less continuous than men's but more continuous than white women (Gibson, 1983; Gibson, 1987). When the issues of impoverishment are examined solely with reference to gender, however, the plight of black men is ignored or understated. It is true that women have a higher incidence of poverty than men of the same race; however, this generalization does not hold across races (Burnham, 1985; Sparr, 1986). For example, poverty rates for African American men are nearly double that for white women. Furthermore, for those African American women who continue to hold jobs, being employed full-time, on a year-round basis is no guarantee against poverty (Higginbotham, 1986).

With these huge wage differentials, which have major implications for retirement income, drawing on strengths and using preventive techniques become important for economic security in later life. These will be addressed in the latter section of this chapter.

Retirement

Prior to the 20th century, retirement as we know it did not exist (Blank, 1982). As large-scale businesses and organizations began to rise in the late 19th century, the meaning of property was altered. The circumstances and motivations of economic activity, as well as the careers and expectations of most citizens, were affected. The resulting bureaucratic principle of efficiency led to the discharge of employees after a certain age, with mandatory retirement policies being the by-product (Achenbaum, 1978).

Retirement has many components and can be rather complex. There is considerable public debate about the full range of consequences of retirement and even some disagreement about the term *retirement*. Everyone experiencing it reacts differently, some greeting it with eager anticipation and loving it, others dreading it, with great variation between these points. For low-income wage earners, retirement is often a luxury they can ill afford.

Retirement is a generalized social pattern, institutionally sanctioned and occurring when people live long enough, the economy can withstand their transition from worker to nonworker status, and social insurance of some form is available (Atchley, 1976). Economic incentives for retirement come in the form of Social Security benefits, private pension funds, profit-sharing, and annuities (Blau, 1984; Coyle, 1984). Because of interrupted work patterns, low-level working status, occupationally segregated jobs, and discrimination, women's preparedness for economic security during retirement is less than that of men (Perkins, 1992, 1993a).

Retirement is a process that begins long before the last day of work and continues well after the good-byes to co-workers are expressed (Atchley, 1976). Atchley states that "Retirement...refers primarily to the final phase of the occupation life cycle..." (p. 1). Generally, one is considered retired if he or she is not working full-time and derives a large portion of financial support from public or private pension payments (Hendricks, & Hendricks, 1981).

Retirement can take several continuous and overlapping forms, the most common being voluntary vs. involuntary, early vs. on-time, and partial vs. complete (Atchley, 1976). Voluntary retirement implies that the worker has made a choice to terminate work and enjoy income derived from an extended period of prior employment. Involuntary retirement is defined as leaving the work force earlier than anticipated (Perkins, 1994).

Retirement involves three major periods—preretirement, transition, and postretirement. The preretirement period typically involves looking ahead to a future life. It is a period during which decisions about whether and when to retire are made (Atchley, 1982). If economic security in retirement is to be realized, it is during the preretirement period that planning must occur (Hall, 1980; Hayes & Deren, 1990).

Preretirement planning (PRP) is probably the single most formidable means of prevention against postretirement hardship known to many older adults. It can help to insure economic, social, and psychological well-being in late life. Unfortunately, PRP is a concept that has not been vastly utilized by older Americans over the last two decades. The greatest barrier to people obtaining PRP is availability. Retirement planning programs typically have not existed in most firms and companies until very recently (Perkins, 1994). Where PRP programs do exist, encouraging older workers to take advantage of them has been met with limited success. This is most likely due to the fears associated with retirement, that is, loss of status, growing old, impending death, and so forth (Perkins, 1994).

The retirement phase traditionally involves a life period without an income-producing job, along with probable changes in health, activity, or living arrangements (Atchley, 1982b). Retirement income is usually decreased to that of about one-half to one-third of a person's former wages. Working class people obviously receive a lower retirement income (Atchley, 1982a; Perkins, 1993a). Almost twice as many men than women over age 65 receive private pension income related to their own work record (46% vs. 23.5%) (Perkins, 1994). In 1991, the average yearly pension benefit for men over 65 was $7,059 compared to $3,647 for women (Leonard, 1994). African American older women, in general, receive lower Social Security benefits than white older women and are only half as likely as their white counterparts to receive a private pension (Gould, 1989; Perkins 1993a). The total monthly Social Security benefit for African American women age 65 to 69 in 1992 averaged $467. For white women, it was $512 (Social Security Administration, 1993).

Much has been written on life satisfaction and quality of life in postretirement. Both depend on the individual's personality, income, health, social circumstances, and sense of worth. Probably health and income are the more predominant predictors of quality of life, with the working-class being the most adversely effected by these two factors.

Women outlive men and, therefore, will have a higher representation in retirement than men. In 1990 there were 67.3 men for every 100 women (U.S. Bureau of the Census, 1990). Retirement is different for women than it is for men. Marital status, living arrangements, and physical health are factors that have an influence on how older women live. Marital status impacts the financial condition of every woman and necessarily impacts on the type of housing that each can afford. African American women are more likely than white women to have never married or, if married, to be separated or divorced, and they have a greater likelihood of being widowed (Gould, 1989). Affordable health care is also a critical problem for poor women since they are highly dependent on employment and marital status for health care benefits. Four to five million older women spend much of their Social Security payments for health care (Stone, 1986). All the prevention (i.e., preretirement planning) one can muster may not be enough to avert some of these inherent, institutionalized conditions facing women in retirement; nonetheless, awareness cannot hurt.

Just what is prevention and what can be expected from it? In the strict sense of the word, it means to keep a thing from happening. Loosely defined, for the purpose of this chapter, it will be defined more as an intervention. Rather than long-term, preplanned prevention, it will be used in the context of short-term prevention and intervention on a daily, weekly, monthly, and yearly basis. Prevention-intervention will be addressed not only as it relates to individuals but also at the community level. It needs to be placed in perspective as well; which prevention-interventions might be best for which person or group? The overall focus will be on strengths and empowerment, with the end result being lower stress and anxiety and good mental health. This goal will be approached from several different aspects, using both traditional and nontraditional concepts: work (paid and unpaid), volunteerism, support groups, peer counseling, play, religion/spirituality, and tapping community resources.

Learning to Use Leisure Time

As discussed in preceding chapters, feelings of loneliness, boredom, and isolation can lead to stress and poor mental health. It is not necessarily the advent of retirement and all that accompanies it, including an abundance of leisure time, that produces these feelings. However, it may be a contributing factor.

There are as many ways to fill the leisure time that employment once occupied as there are individuals; some do it with ease, others struggle. People who have never traveled or developed inwardly by engaging in satisfying hobbies prior to their 60s usually have a difficult time when they first try to "enjoy their leisure" (Meyer, 1980, p. 66). It takes learning and practice to acquire the necessary skills to travel easily and pleasurably or to play authentically so that hobbies and other activities can be genuinely satisfying rather than a time killer (Meyer, 1980).

Mental health programs have long been grappling with the underutilization of formal services to assist older adults to cope with stress. Mental health providers in the 1980s generated many creative programs to deal with this underutilization (c.f. Hult, 1980; Meyer, 1980; Ross, 1983; Sargent, 1980), each with strong empowerment components. Some of these programs will be discussed in this chapter, demonstrating how the strengths model can be applied to this end.

SELF-ACTUALIZATION AND EMPOWERMENT

When looking for ways to reach underserved older adults, Meyer (1980) was stimulated by Maslow's method of studying the well-adjusted rather than the maladjusted. To accomplish this, Meyer sought out community resources. She identified a group of older adults who were leading meaningful and zestful lives and asked them how they were doing it. The result was the formulation of a New Directions Workshop Program designed to help older adults who were having difficulty with the transition into the freedom of their senior years. Through the Program workshops she worked with older adults to set new goals for themselves and to provide the support necessary for them to achieve their goals.

Meyer's program embraces several of the components of the strengths model: empowerment, dialogue and collaboration, membership, synergy and regeneration. The strengths perspective strives to discover the power within people rather than returning power to people. Collaboration occurs when the social worker becomes the client's agent, consultant, or stakeholder in whatever projects or goals that are undertaken. In a collaborative relationship, the social worker and the client seek to discover the individual and community resources that will best facilitate the achievement of the client's wants or goals. When the person and the community come together, synergy occurs. Synergy between the client and social worker occurs when there is a relationship based on reciprocity, a common purpose, and joint recognition of the community as a resource. This subsequently leads to membership and then to regeneration. Community and people are both used as resources. Figures 8.1 and 8.2 use Meyer's program to illustrate the use of the strengths model to empower people via the community.

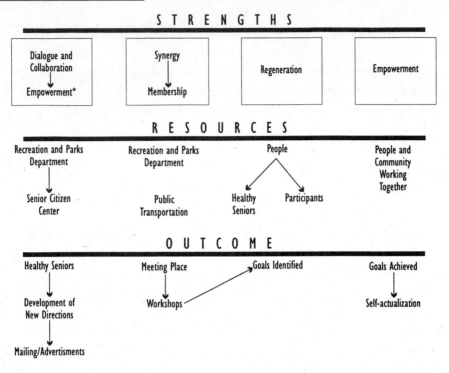

STRENGTHS

| Dialogue and Collaboration ↓ Empowerment* | Synergy ↓ Membership | Regeneration | Empowerment |

RESOURCES

| Recreation and Parks Department ↓ Senior Citizen Center | Recreation and Parks Department ↓ Public Transportation | People ↙ ↘ Healthy Seniors Participants | People and Community Working Together |

OUTCOME

| Healthy Seniors ↓ Development of New Directions ↓ Mailing/Advertisments | Meeting Place ↓ Workshops | Goals Identified | Goals Achieved ↓ Self-actualization |

*A process by which people are empowered through the empowerment of community resources; macro to micro.

FIGURE 8.1 *Community strengths as a resource*

Community as Resource

As seen in Figure 8.1, the strengths of the community were assessed and utilized. Collaboration took place with community resources as well as individuals. The end result was the achievement of a group of individuals' goals. The Senior Citizen Center, housed in a Recreation and Parks Department facility, was utilized to locate older adults living full and happy lives who were willing to be interviewed. The interview study was used to help design the New Directions Workshop Program. The Recreation and Parks Department also supplied the meeting space to hold the workshops and the advertisement necessary to reach prospective participants. The location of the center was such that participants could use public transportation.

People as Resources

In developing the program, a process was provided that offered mutual support for older adults. Initially, the process began with the interviews of the seniors at the Senior Citizen Center. Next, the workshops were developed, offering a variety of programs that focused on people working together to choose, define, and achieve goals. The first goal of the workshop was to develop a trusting atmosphere for the group. The second was to develop awareness that new directions were available and to arouse hope and confidence, and the third was to choose a goal and begin to take steps toward its realization. Figure 8.2 shows how the strengths model is applied, demonstrating how prevention/intervention is taken from the macro- to microlevels of practice. The process is seen as cyclical, beginning and ending with dialogue and collaboration. A collaboration relationship is necessary for both macro and micro practice whereby the practitioner/social worker and the client seek to discover the individual and communal resources that will best facilitate the achievement of the client's wants or goals (Weick, Rapp, Sullivan, & Kisthardt, 1989).

A basic issue emerging from the workshops was the need of the older adults to move beyond the work ethic values of the middle years. It was determined that new yardsticks were needed for measuring what makes

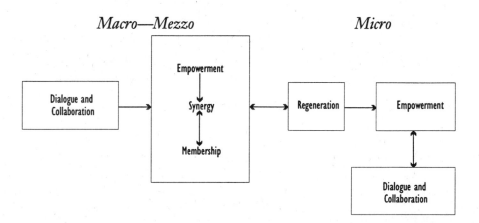

FIGURE 8.2 *Strengths concepts on a continum from macro to micro. Prevention/intervention is shown to be cyclical using strengths components to guide the process.*

life worth living. Again Meyer drew on Maslow, seeing that persever-ance, industriousness, competence, and achievement are splendid val-ues but are not enough. The expression of growth needs included in Maslow's theory of self-actualization requires the development of other virtues as well. For example, the cultivation of aliveness, individuality, playfulness, effortlessness, goodness, and meaningfulness seem espe-cially appropriate during the senior years. This was done with the recognition that while self-actualization is the ideal, it is not always the case for older adults. The freedom and leisure, however, of senior years can provide the conditions for more self-actualization to occur. In the strengths vernacular, self-actualization equates to empowerment.

CASE EXAMPLE

Adell sought out the New Directions workshops within one month of her retirement. Adell, age 68, had just retired from a rigorously sched-uled job as a court reporter with some apprehensions. "I must confess, I'm a little worried about money now that my income has dropped to less than half. And, spending so much time at home with Bert (her husband), gosh, that will seem strange." He had retired several years earlier and had urged Adell to retire so that they could have more time together. Adell said, "Bert is quite relaxed and comfortable in retire-ment but I have to tell you I disapprove of his easy-going attitude and worry that I might become as disorganized and casual about life as he has." Adell defined her initial goals almost in haste: She did not want to become disorganized, and she wanted to take a part-time job to finance travel. Through support and permission from the workshop group she attenuated these early goals and began to express interest in the local community college, deciding to enroll in some classes as a start toward her new direction. She said, "The acting classes really jump out at me but I feel like I ought to do something more educational, like maybe philosophy, instead. And what about a schedule? I still need time to get my other work done."

In group she got in touch with some fears. "Gosh, I don't know if I can do this. It has been so long since I've been in school. What if I don't do well, or what if I get bored?" Through group support, she came to see that she had the right to drop courses if she didn't like them. She signed up for the acting class, which she thoroughly enjoyed, and actually ended up doing less work in other classes and feeling comfortable about this.

After two quarters of classes, she became less enthralled with college and began to put her life in balance on a broader and more self-actualized basis. She took a part-time job (8 hours per week) saying, "I didn't realize how strongly I felt about having a paycheck, even if it isn't much. I still want more than this though. Right now I feel like I'm just filling time. All those years stuck in court listening to people's problems, I longed to do something to help. Now seems like the time." She began by volunteering her services in a booth at the local mall representing the Retired Seniors Volunteer Program (RSVP), in spite of some earlier misgivings about her adequacy for the job. Once again, the group encouraged her in pursuing this endeavor. After gaining some confidence, she left RSVP and she and her husband volunteered at the Meals on Wheels program where they jointly worked one day a week delivering meals. They set aside one day weekly for tennis or golf. The couple then enlarged their service sphere to include monthly outings with a group of teenage girls with developmental disabilities and were adopted as their surrogate grandparents. Adell said, "I felt we were on a roll so why not, and besides we were having so much fun, it's all so rewarding" (Meyer, 1980).

Adell was able to work through her anxiety about what to do with her leisure time. At one level, there was the probable prevention of discord within and possible deterioration of her marriage by early intervention as well as preventing the possible onslaught of her own depression. At another level, there was supportive maintenance of adequate social relationships through the group interaction at the workshops. Still, at other levels, avocational counseling, self-actualization and empowerment came into play (Meyer, 1980).

OTHER APPROACHES FOR PREVENTION/INTERVENTION

Another 1980s project, the Neighborhood Family Project, centered around the empowering concept of neighborhood and family. The driving force behind this unique project was the premise that a major source of stress for older adults is a sense of powerlessness over their destiny. This project went directly to the community of older adults they wanted to reach. The project was called Neighborhood Family (NF) (Ross, 1983).

Like Meyer's program, this project embraced the strengths model's components of empowerment, dialogue and collaboration, membership, synergy, and regeneration. The organizers designed the project so that the decision-making roles, management positions, control of operations, and caring peer support all grew out of the participants' efforts. This approach not only taps individual and community strengths that lead to empowerment; it promotes membership and synergy, which leads to regeneration of the person as well as the environment (community).

The design of this project was fundamentally in keeping with the tenets set forth by McKnight (1992). One of McKnight's concerns was that professional intervention tends to isolate people from their informal community supports. It is not possible to call services for people community services if they do not involve people in community relationships. McKnight (1992) made a distinction between local services and community services. For example, there can be a relocation of services to local places with almost no positive effect on the participation of labeled persons in the community.

The labeled persons in this chapter are isolated older adults. McKnight (1992) recommends that community guides, rather than professionals, be used to help integrate new programs (or persons) into a community. The evolution of the NF was rooted in the community itself, using the geographic residents from the beginning to help put the program in place. This direct participation of the residents served to prevent the isolation from community supports that McKnight suggested occurs when professionals intervene.

The name of the project, Neighborhood Family, was selected to enlist individuals from an area that they themselves defined, psychologically as well as geographically, as their neighborhood and for the bonding values and relationships implied by the term family. The term family was chosen to counter the defensive wariness and social isolation often found among older people who have either lost their friendship networks or kinship base. This premise allowed older people to adopt a surrogate family in order to replace the ties of natural succor and concern formerly provided by the biological family. The actual organization within a specific neighborhood ensured easy access to a resource center and meeting place, common environmental problems, realistic boundaries for community action, and a psychological home base for supportive and outreach activities (Ross, 1983).

The community was tapped by actually canvasing neighborhoods to locate high concentrations of older people. The project's first facility was an old decrepit warehouse (rent free). The older persons who had been recruited painted and refurbished the warehouse making it a warm and attractive meeting place. After the facility was secured, the organization of the seniors and services began. In the beginning, the older people who attended came mostly to satisfy their curiosity, because they had nothing better to do, or because they had a problem. This was a test-the-water phase, and gradually the people gained more and more direct interest. The seniors sponsored an open house designed to introduce the NF to the community and brought residents together with representatives of major community agencies. After the open house, membership expanded and the family concept was readily assimilated by older persons hungry for social outlets and peer supports (Ross, 1983).

As seen in Figure 8.3, the model skips the mezzo level and goes directly to the macro level, the community, for the people it wishes to serve. In this way the community is the power base from which the people become empowered or self-actualized.

The center was staffed by a mental health gerontologist, a nurse, a social worker, and a part-time psychiatrist. The NF was conceived as a coming together, like a family, for the purpose of mutual assistance. The NF was deliberately understaffed in order to encourage development of management skills by the membership. Members were specifically oriented toward assuming responsibility for each other as a surrogate family, and members were encouraged to take part in the

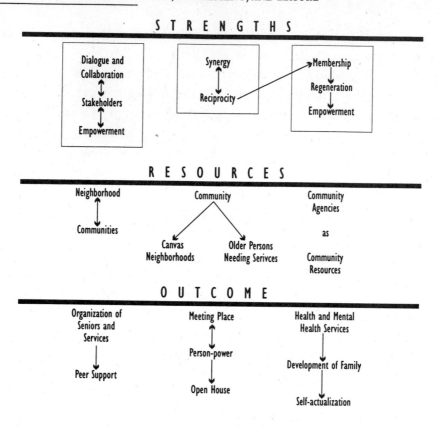

FIGURE 8.3 *The strengths of people within the community: Birth of the neighborhood family. The people in the community are directly accessed, with the community serving as the power base by which people are empowered; the macro and micro become interchangable.*

political process and in community development activities so that they could deal with environmental stressors such as crime, poor sanitation, and other problems in their own neighborhood. With this NF model, the staff provided older people with mental health and medical services while the seniors themselves served as a support group for each other (Ross, 1983).

The NF model used a holistic multidisciplinary service approach with the members. While the staff assumed the single responsibility of making sure that the community and hospital service reached the unwell members, member-senior companions were assigned to home-bound NF members. Additional services were provided for members in the hospital or at home.

Ross (1983) provided an example:

> A member brought in her 65-year-old female neighbor for financial assistance and "because she screams at night and keeps me up." The new member was depressed, agitated, and in a state of confusion. Her appearance was disheveled and dirty. She had stopped taking medication dispensed by a hospital psychiatric outpatient clinic on the advice of her neighbors who convinced her that "the pills" caused all her problems.
>
> In the past 1 ½ years, the woman had experienced 20 admissions to a psychiatric hospital with an underlying diagnosis of chronic undifferentiated schizophrenia and multiple other psychiatric diagnoses. Hospital stays lasted from 1 week to 3 months.
>
> The NF psychiatrist stabilized the woman's symptoms with appropriate psychotropic medication. The nurse and social worker helped her to achieve her goals (financial assistance, referral and follow along for medical differential diagnosis, improved housing, and "to see my family"). Initially she was withdrawn and frightened, but this subsided with members' encouragement. They also monitored her drug and medical regime, provided companionship to her in the evening, and directed the procedure for successfully reestablishing contact with her family, whom she had not seen for 20 years. Socialization increased slowly as her behavior, appearance, and outlook improved. When she was rejected by a male NF participant, members helped her through this crisis and others by their continuous support and availability. In her second year with the program, she contributed her piano talents to a NF singing group and, in turn, received valued peer recognition. She refused to accept a new apartment in a housing project because it was "too far from the family." In the ensuing years, the woman underwent no further hospitalizations. (From "The Neighborhood Family: Community Mental Health for the Elderly," by H. K. Ross, 1983, *Gerontologist, 23* (3), 246.)

This may seem like an extreme case. However, it is a good example of how working with a person's strengths can enable and empower them to take control of their lives. The strong sense of community the NF provided for this woman gave her back her membership in an otherwise hostile environment. The encouragement and support from other "family" members gave her the courage to take some risks in terms of self-care and expanding her horizons. It did take some time, but by her second year as a NF family member her mental health stabilized sufficiently that she could make her own decisions and actually venture into a world of living fully rather than merely existing. The synergy that occurred between her and the community led to a regeneration process.

Peer Counseling

Peer counseling is another form of prevention where people help each other. Its uniqueness lies in the fact that trained women and men who are not professionals work with persons of similar age and experience. It has special appeal for older people who are reluctant to seek out professional services. The peer counseling concept facilitates the establishment of a special rapport that allows genuine supportive relationships to develop (Bratter & Tuvman, 1980).

Volunteering

In the aging community, older volunteers are used specifically to provide human contact to other older people who are confined and isolated. These volunteers consist of neighborhood or organizational support networks, for example, Retired Senior Volunteer Program (RSVP), senior services centers, councils on aging, nutrition programs, day-care and day-activity centers, and health and recreational programs. These in turn have generated other programs with more focused therapeutic potential, such as homemaker services, home health services, senior companion programs, friendly visiting, or a number of telephone reassurance projects (Hult, 1980).

In addition to the benefits of volunteering for isolated older persons, it also fills a need for the older volunteer. In a study done by Tinsley, Colbs, Teaff, and Kaufman (1987) on the psychological benefits of leisure activities for older persons, a high percentage of respondents listed volunteerism as a satisfying leisure activity: 67% for men, 45% for women.

Computer Technology

Senior Net is a national computer program accessible to older adults who have computers and to senior centers with computers. Not only does it provide the challenge of acquiring computer skills, it is recreational, educational, and can be lifesaving. An older women, Eileen, who lived alone in North Carolina, suffered a stroke and was able to get to her computer and send an SOS message to her computer counterparts in another state who were able to get her immediate help. She said of Senior Net, "I love it, I'm right up there with them (youngsters), I'm 'surfing' on my keyboard" (Davis, 1995).

Innovations for Older Workers in the Marketplace

Some older people return to work after retirement out of economic necessity. Others seek personal satisfaction out of paid employment. Whatever the reason, paid work can be seen as prevention-intervention for older adults in the form of added financial security and as an aid to ward off poor mental health. Perkins (1994) listed some innovative work options for older people wanting employment.

Banks With a lifetime of managing their money, older workers excel as tellers and customer-service representatives. The Bank of America in Los Angeles provides two weeks of training and typically pays $7 to $10 an hour.

Hotels In 1985, two Days Inns found that the average employee quit after three months; this was accompanied by an absentee rate of 30%. Days Inn tapped the over-55 labor market, and today, in nearly a third of the centers, 450 employees are 55 or older. Their average tenure is three years; the absentee rate is 3%; the average salary is $6.50 an hour.

Hardware stores Picture yourself roaming a hardware store in search of the right widget to fix the toilet. A mature face suggests years of fix-up experience to you. This is a lesson learned by home-improvement chains like Builders Emporium, (where 15% of the 6,200 employees are over age 55), as well as Hechinger and Home

Depot. A typical salary in a California Builders Emporium is $7.35 per hour.

Most older people require some retraining in order to step into the dignified and healthy jobs that will help sustain them financially. Few programs specifically provide retraining for older adults. An exception is the program Senior Community Services Employment (SCSE), which is funded by the Older Americans Act of 1965. This program provides part-time subsidized employment opportunities for older adults, making a difference both in their income and quality of life (Mor-Barak & Tynan, 1993; Perkins, 1994).

There are other programs that draw on public and community resources and, to some extent, private industry. These programs for older workers typically fall into two categories. One facilitates linkages between older adults and potential employers. The other accommodates the needs of older adults in the workplace through job modification, job training, and senior care. For a full description of these programs see Mor-Barak and Tynan (1993) and Perkins (1994).

RELIGION AND SPIRITUALITY

While not considered a prevention program per se, religion and spirituality play an important role in the lives of most older adults in helping to promote good mental health. Maslow's view of human potential gradually expanded and he added a higher need level which he labeled self-transcendence. This manifested from his belief that human beings have a longing to transcend aloneness and feel a connection to others and to the cosmos (Maslow, 1968). The more years that people live, the greater the experiences they will have to reflect on, the greater the hunger they will have to explain themselves to themselves, and the deeper their need will be to justify their existence on the Earth (Vayhinger, 1980).

Over the past two hundred years, the relationship between the church and state has changed drastically. The government has gradually taken over many functions that religious institutions had once performed. These changes, however, have been less profound in the older adult population. Places of worship have continued to care for and express concern for older persons. Likewise, seniors have maintained far greater involvement with religion than with other social institutions (Vayhinger, 1980).

Whether or not an older person holds a specific religious belief, many have some connection with spirituality or have spiritual needs that beg to be addressed, especially as they approach death. From an earlier White House Conference on Aging, Moberg (1971, cited in Vayhinger, 1980) identified six areas of spiritual need: (a) sociocultural needs, (b) relief from anxieties and fears, (c) a philosophy of life, (d) personality integration, (e) freedom from personal disunity, and (f) preparation for death.

Vayhinger (1980) expressed the concern of older adults regarding death as follows:

> Death attitudes are complex, depending upon the depth and intensity of the particular beliefs of the persons involved; the person may feel "forgiven" or "saved" or "close to God," may be aware of approaching death, may feel supported by the presence of the clergy and family, etc. (p. 206)

Not all social workers and other mental health providers will feel comfortable or competent in working with older adults in religious or spiritual matters. Most holistic teams, however, now include clergy. If these resources are not available, referrals can be made.

Browning's famous poem seems appropriate here:

> Grow old along with me
> The best is yet to be.
> The last of life for which the first was made:
> Our times are in His hand
> Who saith, "A Whole I planned.
> Trust God, see all, nor be afraid."

Summary

While there are sure to be many other innovative approaches to prevention/intervention regarding mental health issues for older adults, the examples provided in this chapter give the reader an overview of a wide range of such services along with examples demonstrating how to integrate the strengths concepts into existing programs. Figures 8.1, 8.2, and 8.3 provide graphic descriptions that can be translated and applied to new programs.

This chapter shows that, in terms of prevention, clinical interventions are not always necessary. Alternative approaches that draw on the strengths of communities and people are integral components to mental health intervention/prevention when working with older adults.

REFERENCE

Achenbaum, A. (1978). *Old age in the new land*. Baltimore, MD: Johns-Hopkins University Press.

Atchley, R. (1976). *The sociology of retirement*. New York: Schenkman.

Atchley, R. (1982a). Retirement: Leaving the world of work. *The Annals of the American Academy of Policy and Social Science, 464*, 120–131.

Atchley, R. (1982b). The process of retirement: Comparing women and men. In M. Szinovacz (Ed.), *Women's retirement: Policy implications of recent research* (pp. 41–56). Beverly Hills, CA: Sage Publications.

Bergmann, B. (1971). The effect on white incomes of discrimination in employment. *Journal of Political Economy, 79*, 294–313.

Blank, R. (1982). A changing work life and retirement pattern: An historical prospective. In M. Morrison (Ed.), *Economics of aging: The future of retirement* (pp. 1–60). New York: Van Nostrand Reinhold Company.

Blau, F. (1984). Occupational segregation and labor market discrimination. In B. F. Reskin (Ed.), *Sex segregation in the workplace: trends, explanations, remedies* (pp. 117–143). Washington, DC: National Academy Press.

Bratter, B., and Tuvman, E. (1980). A peer counseling program in action. In S.S. Sargent (Ed.), *Nontraditional therapy and counseling with the aging* (pp. 131–145). New York: Springer Publishing Co.

Burnham, L. (1985). Has poverty been feminized in Black America? *The Black Scholar, 16*, 14–24.

Cory, E. (1993, June 10). Report on women's salaries. *Morning Edition*. Washington, DC: National Public Radio.

Coyle, J. M. (1984). Women's attitudes toward planning for retirement. *Convergence, 2*, 120–131.

Daniel, P. (1994, September/October). Learning to love growing old. *Psychology Today*, 61–70.

Davis, K. (1995, January 25). Report on Senior Net Services. *Morning Edition.* Washington, DC: National Public Radio.

England, P., & Farkas, G. (1986). *Households, employment, and gender.* New York: Aldine Publishing Co.

Erikson, E. H. (1963). *Childhood and society* (2nd ed.). New York: W.W. Norton and Co.

Faludi, S. (1991). *Backlash: The undeclared war against American women.* New York: Crown Publishing, Inc.

Gibson, R. (1983). *Work and retirement: Aging black women—a race and sex comparison.* (Final report to the Administration on Aging). Ann Arbor, MI: The University of Michigan.

Gibson, R. (1987). Reconceptualizing retirement for Americans. *The Gerontologist, 27* (6), 691–698.

Gould, K. H. (1989). A minority-feminist perspective on women and aging. In J.D. Garner & S.O. Mercer (Eds.), *Women as they age: Challenge, opportunity, and triumph* (pp. 195–216). New York: The Haworth Press, Inc.

Hall G. (1980, Summer). Retirement planning: Suggestions for management. *Aging and Work,* 203-209.

Hayes, C. L. & Deren, J. M. (1990). *Pre-retirement planning for women: Program design and research.* New York: Springer Publishing Co.

Hendricks, J. & Hendricks, C. D. (1981). *Aging in mass society: Myths and realities* (2nd ed.). Cambridge, MA: Winthrop.

Higgenbotham, E. (1986). We were never on a pedestal: Women of color continue to struggle with poverty, racism, and sexism. In R. Lefkowitz & A. Withorn (Eds.), *For crying out loud* (pp. 97–108). New York: Pilgrim Press.

Hult, H. (1980). The volunteer connection. In S. S. Sargent (Ed.), *Nontraditional therapy and counseling with the aging* (pp. 119–130). New York: Springer Publishing Co.

Levitan, S., Mangum, G., & Marshall, R. (1976). *Human resources and labor markets* (2nd ed.). New York: Harper and Row.

Madden, J. F. (1985). The persistence of pay differentials: The economics of sex discrimination. In L. Larwood, S. Stromberg, & B. Gutek (Eds.), *Women and Work.* Beverly Hills, CA: Sage Publications.

Maslow, A. (1968). *Toward a psychology of being.* New York: Van Nostrand Reinhold Co.

McKnight, J. (1992). Redefining community. *Social Policy, 23,* 56–62.

Meyer, G. (1980). The new directions workshop for Senior Citizens. In S.S. Sargent (Ed.), *Nontraditional therapy and counseling with the aging* (pp. 55–73). New York: Springer Publishing Co.

Mor-Barak, M. E., & Tynan, M. (1993). Older workers and the workplace: A new challenge for occupational social work. *Social Work, 38*(1), 45–55.

National Commission on Working Women. (1986, Spring/Summer). *Women at Work, 3*, p. 2.

Older Women's League. (1986, May). *Report on the status of midlife and older women.* Washington, DC: Author.

Older Women's League. (1990). *Heading for hardship: Retirement income for American women in the next century.* Washington, DC: Author.

Perkins, K. (1992). Psychosocial implications of women and retirement. *Social Work, 37*(6), 526–532.

Perkins, K. (1993a) Working-class women and retirement. *Journal of Gerontological Social Work, 20*(1).

Perkins, K. (1993b). Recycling poverty: From the workplace to retirement. *Journal of Women and Aging, 5*(1), 5–23.

Perkins, K. (1994). Older women in the workplace and implications for retirement: EAP can make a difference. *Employment Assistance Quarterly, 9*(3/4), 81–97.

Ross, H. K. (1983). The neighborhood family: Community mental health for the elderly. *The Gerontologist, 23*(3), 243–247.

Sargent, S. S. (1980). *Nontraditional therapy and counseling with the aging.* New York: Springer Publishing Co.

Smith, J., & Ward, M. (1984). *Women's wages and work in the twentieth century.* Santa Monica, CA: Rand Publishers.

Social Security Administration. (1993). Annual Statistical Supplement. *Social Security Bulletin.* Washington, DC: Author.

Sparr, P. (1986). Reevaluating feminist economics: "Feminization of poverty" ignores key issues. In R. Lefkowitz & A. Withorn (Eds.), *For crying out loud* (pp. 61–66). New York: Pilgrim Press.

Stone, R. (1986). *The feminization of poverty and older women: An update.* Washington, DC: National Center for Health Services Research.

Tinsley, H. E. A., Colbs, S. L., Teaff, J. D., & Kaufman, N. (1987). The relationship of age, gender, health and economic status to the psychological benefits older persons report from participation in leisure activities. *Leisure Sciences, 9*, 53–65.

U.S. Bureau of Census. (1990). *General population characteristics.* Washington, DC: U.S. Department of Commerce, Economics, and Statistics Administration.

U.S. Bureau of Census. (1992). *Poverty in the United States: 1992.* Consumer Income, Series P60-185. Washington, DC: U.S. Department of Commerce, Economics, and Statistics Administration.

U.S. Bureau of Census. (1994). *Statistical Abstract of the United States, 1994*. Washington, DC: U.S. Department of Commerce, Economics, and Statistics Administration.

Vayhinger, J. M. (1980). The approach of pastoral psychology. In S.S. Sargent (Ed.), *Nontraditional therapy and counseling with the aging* (pp. 199–213). New York: Springer Publishing Co.

Weick, A., Rapp, C., Sullivan, P. W., & Kishardt, W. (1989). A strengths perspective for social work practice. *Social Work, 34*, 350–354.

CHAPTER NINE

Long-term Care from a Strengths Perspective

MANY OF THE THEMES AND RESEARCH related to older adults focus on issues of long-term care, the medical and social interventions that support persons with chronic conditions. Similar to health care, long-term care involves a continuum of services in an array of sites ranging from the community to residential facilities. Vital to sustaining quality life, long-term care highlights the nation's position that old age is a personal problem requiring private solutions. Nowhere else in the world are expectations for care so clearly defined as the responsibility of older people, their families, and informal systems of support (Olson, 1994; Kane & Kane, 1976).

Since the United States has not developed a comprehensive policy for long-term care, the quality and option of services available to a particular individual primarily depends on personal economic resources and family members as caregivers. The American sense of individual-ism and self-reliance presupposes older adults will support their social, financial, and service needs. In the context of purchase of services, the government is the provider of last resort with the Medicaid program providing nearly all funding for long-term care. Consequently, publicly supported long-term care, in the form of either home-based services or nursing homes, are provided primarily to older people without family systems of support, who have experienced poverty throughout their lives or are newly impoverished.

This chapter explores how the strengths model relates to long-term care for older adults with mental health challenges. Redefining the nation's response to demand for long-term care necessitates a change in focus from how well individuals use long-term services to how well individuals are actually functioning in long-term care. In this approach, the effectiveness of the long-term care system is measured according to each person's definition of successful community living. Practically, this approach involves a high degree of individualization that usually does not exist in most systems-level research. However, this appears to be a relevant way to measure the success of long-term care in terms of its actual impact on the lives of older adults.

Approaches to Long-term Care

The current demand for long-term care reflects an aging population, the increased prevalence of the oldest-old subgroup with high risks of functional and cognitive challenges, including Alzheimer's disease, and the delay of mortality (Mechanic, 1989). How the nation responds to individuals with long-term care needs corresponds to societal beliefs and values. The majority of long-term services fall into three broad categories defined by where services are provided and by whom.

FAMILY SERVICES

Research indicates that American families provide approximately 80% of all long-term care in the United States. Morris and Morris (1994) stated that for every older adult in a nursing home, there are at least three to as many as five comparable adults in the community. Of the people at risk for facility placement, less than one in five will enter a nursing home. Older adults remain in the community, with chronic health conditions and diminishing cognitive abilities, due to a network of complex and continuing services.

During the past 25 years, informal support systems, primarily family members, have assumed the critical sustaining role. Shanas's (1979) work remains relevant: Older people remain in the community primarily because of the dedicated work of relatives and friends. Juster's (1993) Health and Retirement Survey concluded middle-aged Americans not only care for their aging parents rather than abandon them but consider caregiving a family obligation rather than a burden.

To supplement family services, some older adults pay professionals for components of long-term care, including chore services, homemaking services, nursing care, and physical therapy. The length of service use depends largely on the person's physical condition and financial resources. Even with the purchase of services, most frail older adults tend to rely on families and, to varying degrees, friends for some portion of their care (Stone, Cafferata, & Sangl, 1987).

Most often, family services are the responsibility of one family member who delivers actual care and coordinates a network of supports. Women represent 70% of all caregivers, including adult daughters (30%), spouses (23%), and other women relatives, many of whom are daughters-in-law and sisters (20%). Husbands provide 13% of total care, followed by sons (9%), and other male relatives (7%) (Olson, 1994; Brody, 1990).

Caring for an older person is generally an unanticipated role for families. For example, Maggie Louis recalled her response to news of her father: "I was surprised when my father called from the hospital to tell me he had fallen and broken his hip. Although I had gradually accepted being middle-aged, it was difficult to image my father as aging and dependent. The question was, 'Where do we go from here?'"

Abel (1989) found that very few women were emotionally prepared for the role as caregiver to their parents. In particular, child-care needs often complicated caring for parents. To women, caught between children and parents, one of the biggest sources of conflict is deciding who comes first in time allocation. Coupled with the frustration of having multiple obligations is the shock caused by the disease of the aging parent and the suddenness and depth of dependency. However, studies indicate that families prefer to provide care rather than to place their relatives in institutions. In fact, older people are institutionalized primarily as their caregiver becomes exhausted, ill, or dies (Morycz, 1985; Hooyman & Lustbader, 1986).

COMMUNITY-BASED SERVICES

The first response to long-term care needs is family services. Ideally, when family services fall short or are unavailable, the community of service providers responds. As indicated by Table 9.1, a community-based system of long-term care is a coordinated effort to meet the health and social service needs of older adults. Usually organized according to a geographic area, the goal of community services is to assist older people in such a way that they can remain in their private homes. For older persons without a family caregiver, community-based services are particularly significant if a person is to live and remain at home (Roff & Atherton, 1989).

TABLE 9.1   *A Community-based Service System*
              of Long-term Care

SERVICE	GOAL
Home Health Care	To provide a variety of psychological, social, personal, and medical services in an individual's home.
Adult Day Care	To provide socialization, group activities, hot meals, and snacks in group settings.
Adult Day Health Center	To provide medical restorative and supportive services 7 days a week.
Respite	To provide family caregivers with relief from caregiving for a period of time.
Chore Services	To provide specific home management needs including housekeeping, meal preparation, and laundry services.
Meals on Wheels	To provide meals that require minimal or no preparation to individuals in their home.
Assisted Living	To provide assistance with daily activities and monitoring on a 24-hour basis; to provide emergency assistance as needed.

In general, community-based long-term care reflects a haphazard or fragmented approach to services. For example, a person discharged from the hospital after a hip replacement might be involved with several agencies and practitioners to receive services associated with hospitalization discharge and a rehabilitation regime. Coordinating community services is a task in itself. Unfortunately, the result is that older persons often find themselves returning to the hospital or a nursing home because the maze of supportive systems is too difficult to negotiate or the fragmented services leave gaps in necessary care. This was the situation faced by Mrs. Hannah Harper. "I was married for 35 years before my husband died. We never had children, but we lived in our home for over 30 years and we had strong community connections. After my stroke, I wanted to return home and did so for a period of time. But I was unable to manage my care needs and providers. There were so many telephone calls to make and so many different faces and names to keep straight. Receiving care became stressful and slowly my health began to deteriorate. I don't think I would have lived if I didn't move to a nursing home."

During the last decade the national trend has been to institute case management services to coordinate long-term care services. According to Rubin (1992), case management involves an approach to service delivery that "attempts to ensure that people with complex, multiple problems and disabilities received all the services they need in a timely fashion" (p. 5). As a boundary-spanning approach, the function of case management is to link people to direct service providers. By assuming ultimate responsibility for a network of services, case managers assume responsibility for matching a person's needs with appropriate services and monitoring the provision of such services. Usually case managers serve people who remain in their own homes, but case management can be extended to individuals residing in specialized facilities in the absence of other coordinating services.

The success of long-term care community services is based on the continuity and coordination of care, financial resources of the individual, responsiveness of a community service system to a full range of needs, case management services, and willingness of the older person to establish relationships with a variety of service providers. Even if successful, it is doubtful long-term care community services will replace nursing homes because it has not been determined that community services save costs (Olson, 1994; Benjamin, 1985).

Nursing Home Services

Nursing homes flourished after 1965 as a result of Medicare and Medicaid reimbursements. Based on Goffman's (1961) work, Johnson and Grant (1985) concluded that using the term nursing home, "connotes an effort by society to offer a replacement for care and protection by the family" (p. ix). In this context, the long-term care provided by nursing homes represents one end of a continuum of care (Connor, 1992).

The American nursing home tends to reflect a medical model of service with a hospital-like environment and custodial care as the major focus. Under the Omnibus Budget Reconciliation Act of 1987, the traditional pattern of providing services based on levels of care was replaced with care classifications based on the "Index for Levels of Effort" (Barrow, 1992, p. 194). By assessing a set of complex variables related to the facility's care, programs, staff composition, and related factors, a facility is matched with a Level of Effort category. Government reimbursements correspond to each category, and periodic reassessments may result in a facility receiving a higher or lower index.

While it is important to note that only 5% of people 65 years or older spend their last years in nursing homes, 20% of this cohort reside in a long-term care facility for a period of time in their lives (Greenberg, Boyd, & Hale, 1992). Two-thirds of nursing home residents are women, half are 85 years of age or older, and almost half are childless. The vast majority of people have multiple medical problems such as arthritis, diabetes, or heart disease, and they require assistance in the daily activities of living, including eating, dressing, and bathing. From this broad profile, a typical person residing in a nursing home emerges: She is poor, white, widowed, over the age of 80 years, and will remain in long-term care until death.

Many people come to nursing homes from other institutions, such as a medical hospital, with chronic or crippling diagnoses. In either case, the nursing home as a choice for long-term services often depends on a person's level of care and the family's or community's ability to match the care level on a 24-hour basis. From this perspective, nursing is viewed as a specialized resource that is part of an array of services available to an older person.

Unfortunately, if meaningful social activities, psychological care services, or rehabilitative services are provided by nursing homes they are usually a scheduled event rather than an integral part of daily life. People residing in nursing homes are "cast in a sick role where withdrawal from social activities predominate; they are kept both disabled and dependent" (Olson, 1994, p. 38). Although a portion of nursing home residents are challenged by an array of mental health conditions, few facilities provide opportunities for assessment and treatment in the form of individual and/or group counseling.

For example, Mr. George Gotlieb, age 74, needs long-term care. In the last year, his wife of 52 years died. Because of Parkinson's disease, Mr. Gotlieb cannot get out of bed without considerable assistance. His lack of activity has resulted in bedsores. Although Mr. Gotlieb has a son and a daughter, they live several hours away and they both have careers that require considerable travel. Since his admission, Mr. Gotlieb has been withdrawn and often tearful. Mr. Gotlieb refuses to participate in the daily afternoon socialization and recreation activity. He is scheduled to a see a mental health counselor two times monthly, but the last appointment was canceled because of a conflict with his program planning meeting. Mr. Gotlieb's only regular visitor is his rabbi.

Mr. Gotlieb's circumstances reflect several factors associated with long-term care. Specifically, the lack of family caregivers coupled with complicated physical conditions present a complex situation that often forces a person into a long-term care facility. Medication and 24-hour medical supervision often manage physical conditions, but the mental health of people is often neglected or relegated to little active treatment, and this treatment decreases in frequency over time (Shadish, Silber, & Bootzin, 1984).

The provision of care offered Mr. Gotlieb is hampered by a lack of linkages (Bould, Sanborn, & Reif, 1989). Mr. Gotlieb's situation highlights the lack of linkage between his formal and informal support systems, namely, his children, the nursing home staff, his religious leader, and mental health counselor. Also, Mr. Gotlieb's self-determination in relation to choice in activities, mental health needs, and interdependent, reciprocal relationships is not a integral part of the long-term care system.

Moving from the community to a long-term care facility is a decision not easily made. The majority of older adults express a clear preference for remaining at home or at least in the home of a family member. The benefits of remaining at home involve several categories: benefits of independence, benefits related to a neighborhood of social networks, benefits related to home as a nucleus of meaning related to life events and relationships; and benefits of household involvement as exercise for the body and mind (Lawton, 1985; Rowles, 1987; Herzog & House, 1991; Fogel, 1994).

Both older people and their families recognize the importance of home, independent living, and self-determination. As illustrated in Table 9.2, the decision for a person to enter a nursing home often involves conflict and guilt. This inner turmoil results in repeatedly questioning the placement decision and perhaps the selection of the actual nursing home facility. It is not unusual for family members to question whether their role in placement in terms of whether they could have done more to meet their obligations. Thus, for some families the psychological debate is never over. In fact, it often continues throughout the years of nursing home placement.

For three years, Mrs. George lived with her daughter Chris. After Mrs. George experienced a stroke that left her partially paralyzed, Chris realized she could no longer care for her mother at home. The decision was made for nursing home placement. Although Chris visited her mother daily, Mrs. George persistently asked "to go home." Mrs. George died in the nursing home over one year ago; however, Chris continues to wrestle with feelings of guilt that she abandoned her mother.

The questions and concerns associated with Chris and Mrs. George support the notion that nursing homes often have two clients who would benefit from mental health services: the persons in placements *and* their family and friends.

Funding Long-term Care

The major federal programs providing long-term care services were passed by Congress in 1965. These include two programs targeted directly toward the needs of older adults: the Older Americans Act (Act III) and Medicare. Two additional programs, Medicaid and Title XX of the Social Security Act (the Social Services Block Grant Program), were targeted for persons at risk or in need in all age groups (Bould, Sanborn, & Reif, 1989).

The Older Americans Act of 1965 (OAA) contributed to the notion of a continuum of care for older adults. With an emphasis on independence

TABLE 9.2 *Responses to Nursing Home Placement*

	EMOTIONAL REACTION
Older Adults	**Loss**—the feeling of separation from home, family, and friends
	Fear of an unknown environment and people; the feeling that death is approaching
	Depression—an attitude of hopelessness followed by withdrawal, isolation, and inactivity
	Hostility directed to family and care providers who arranged the placement
	Denial of the need for placement and one's physical and mental condition
Family Members	**Guilt** for being unable to provide the necessary care and supervision
	Fear of what the placement means financially and to the family members' physical and mental condition
	Anger toward a failed system of care
	Frustration directed toward the responsibilities and events leading to placement

and individualism, the following OAA objectives are relevant to self-determination for people as they age:

1. The best possible physical and mental health that science can make available, without regard to economic status.

2. Full restorative services for those who require institutional care.

3. Efficient community services, including access to low-cost transportation, which provide a choice in supported living arrangements and social assistance in a coordinated manner and which are readily available when needed.

4. Freedom, independence, and the free exercise of individual initiative in planning and managing their own lives. (U.S. Senate, Special Committee on Aging, 1985a: pp. 1–2)

Amendments to OAA made it even more supportive of a continuum of acute and long-term care. Specifically, the need for in-home care was emphasized and opportunities for self-determination were expanded to avoid premature placements in nursing homes. According to amendments, there was to be "a continuum of care for the vulnerable of the elderly" (U.S. Senate, Special Committee on Aging, 1985a, p. 2). Unfortunately, OAA provided neither the level of funding nor the administrative authority required to attain these objectives. What has developed as a result of OAA is a broad community-based service system, referred to as the aging network comprising information and referral services, transportation, education, nutritional services, and congregate and shared housing (Bould, Sanborn, & Reif, 1989).

Title XX of the Social Security Act was also passed in 1965 and targeted at-risk or in-need older adults for community-based services to prevent unnecessary institutionalization. The federal government provides grants to states for funding Title XX programs, and the majority of states administer programs through local departments of public assistance. The stigma attached to public assistance is a service barrier for older adults, as are income tests, which rate many older persons ineligible or which many people refuse to complete. These issues, coupled with limited funding, have minimized Title XX's potential to fill the gaps of OAA.

Medicare provides acute care services and few resources for long-term care. Consequently, during the last two decades acute medical care has dominated the continuum of services delivered to older adults. In 1965, when the Medicare legislation was passed, physicians and the acute care service system were in operation and were granted a large degree of control of services and resources. By assuming a gatekeeping position, physicians determined the need for help and the caregiving responsibility of families' members. To qualify for personal services under Medicare, an individual must be minimally 65 and in need of skilled care. Custodial services, whether provided at home or in an institution, are not covered by the program. Therefore, most functionally challenged individuals are not served by Medicare.

The Medicaid program is the primary funding source for long-term care. States design and administer the program in compliance with general federal guidelines. Medicaid's original intent was to provide the nation's very poor—primarily single women with children—access to health care. The federal government never intended the program to provide significant amounts of long-term care to older adults. Nevertheless, by 1990, older people represented approximately 20% of the 26 million Medicaid recipients and 40% of the program's total expenditures of $70 billion (Pepper Commission, 1990). According to Olson (1994), "current policy Medicaid expenditures will increase threefold with nursing home fees representing nearly 50% of all costs over the next decade" (p. 29).

Publicly supported institutional care under Medicaid began as a limited response by the government to a relatively small older population. In the 1980s, the demand for long-term care increased far beyond expectations. The increase reflected a growing number of older people turning to Medicaid for reimbursement of nursing home fees. In particular, many middle-income households qualified for Medicaid services after depleting their resources following a year or less of care.

Because of their economic status, older adults with persistent mental health conditions have traditionally been the responsibility of the state. The largest share of their care was provided by government-operated services, namely, the state hospital. The objectives of state hospitals are the objectives of a state's mental health authority. The authority's budget is fixed annually, but its ability to control the volume of people committed to its care is limited. Thus, the state faces considerable pressure to minimize the resources spent on each individual and to reduce the number of people it must serve. As states attempted to shift operating costs to the federal government, older, mentally challenged individuals were transferred from state-funded mental health facilities to nursing homes or other private facilities funded under Medicaid (Hashimi, 1988).

An institutional bias dominates the Medicare and Medicaid programs. This bias translates into approximately three-quarters of the programs' funds allocated to care in hospitals or nursing homes, with most of the remainder allocated to doctors' fees. Further support for the institutional bias came from the Hill-Burton Act, the Small Business Administration, and the Federal Housing Administration mortgage insurance program, which stimulated hospital construction, and later, nursing home construction.

Applying the Model to Long-term Care

America's long-term care system presents three primary challenges for the strengths model of practice. First, the long-term care provided by families, community agencies, or nursing homes signifies a loss of power for older adults, but little attention is paid to the mental health of older adults at any level of care. Second, families provide the majority of in-home services to older adults at an expense to the families' financial, mental, and physical status; however, few mental health services are available for caregivers. Third, society values aging at home in the community, with nursing home services a resource of last resort, but funding sources erode this value with policies that support institutionalization.

Faced with these challenges, social work must consider the strengths model as a practice approach that values prevention as a necessary element for quality of life. In previous chapters, the focus has been on micro issues of social work, those interventions with people in their environments. Considering the strengths model in relation to long-term care involves mezzo and macro practice or social work services with small groups and the larger communities along with the micro aspects of practice.

LOSS OF POWER AND MENTAL HEALTH ISSUES

The key player in any discussion of long-term care is the person in need of services. Although personal losses and a decline in health status are not inevitably associated with aging, older people do experience these conditions at a disproportionately higher rate than does the general population. The strengths model addresses individual loss through a process of empowerment that begins in assessing people in their environments and continues as a unifying thread throughout interventions and evaluations to support the mental health of older adults and their overall quality of life.

For older adults to age in place at home requires that they control the threat of a shrinking life space. According to Cox (1988), as older persons lose strength, experience health losses, and generally begin to feel less in control of their environments, they are likely to restrict their mobility to the areas where they feel secure and welcomed. In comparing older person with other groups, "only small children and those living in institutions are so bound to house and neighborhood" (Cox, 1988, p. 202).

The strengths model enhances the control older adults have over their environments by monitoring four aspects of optimal life conditions, as illustrated in Figure 9.1. By interfacing with these components, concepts of the strengths model ensure that older people maintain control over life even as components change. As indicated by Table 9.3, this is accomplished by considering optimal life conditions in the context of identification of strengths, acceptance of needs and wants, involvement in the change process, and mobilization of resources. Concepts of the strengths model utilize nonmedical premises about aging and differ from traditional approaches in the ways given below.

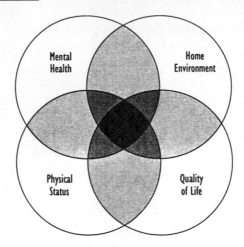

FIGURE 9.1 *Indicators for optimal life conditions*
"Environment and other determinants of well-being in older people," by M. Powell Lawton, 1982, *Gerontologist*, 23, 4, 355.

Older people highlight their strengths. The initial identification of the strengths of older adults set the stage for the rest of all interventions. Building on strengths serves to enhance the mental status of individuals by highlighting their unique values. This is particularly important as people begin to consider their long-term care needs, because for as long as possible, the individuals are recognized as the experts of their lives and anticipated needs. Social workers may offer what they know, have observed, or have been taught, but the final expert on an individual's situation is the older adult.

The social worker recognizes the strength of family members, friends, and the community. From the onset, intervention is viewed as a collaborative effort. Since much of long-term care is provided by family and friends, they must be considered as a source of strength for older adults. Also, the community offers unlimited resources for older adults who define their roles in the context of community.

The social worker does not control the helping process. The strengths model requires that the social worker relinquish the need to control the process and outcome of the intervention with older adults. All actions must be evaluated against the degree to which they enhance

TABLE 9.3 *Optimal Life Conditions Interfaced with the Strengths Model*

| | STRENGTHS MODEL | | | |
OPTIMAL LIFE CONDITIONS	IDENTIFICATION OF STRENGTHS	ACCEPTANCE OF WANTS/ NEEDS	INVOLVEMENT IN CHANGE PROCESS	MOBILIZATION OF RESOURCES
Mental Health	Collaborative assessment	Suspension of disbelief	Membership Synergy Evaluation	Dialogue and collaboration Synergy Regeneration Evaluation
Home Environment	Collaborative assessment Dialogue and collaboration	Suspension of disbelief	Membership Synergy Regeneration Evaluation	Dialogue and collaboration Membership Synergy Regeneration Evaluation
Physical Status	Collaborative assessment Dialogue and collaboration	Suspension of disbelief	Synergy Regeneration Evaluation	Regeneration Dialogue and collaboration
Quality of Life	Collaborative assessment Dialogue and collaboration	Suspension of disbelief	Dialogue and collaboration Membership Synergy Regeneration Evaluation	Dialogue and collaboration Membership Synergy Regeneration Evaluation

the quality of an older person's life as defined by that person. Social workers must avoid "doing for" and "doing to" and learn to take cues from older adults by listening to their definitions of needs and blending the wisdom of age with professional training.

The situations and long-term care needs of older adults belong to the immediate environment and, simultaneously, to a larger arena. Traditional approaches to service delivery view the helping process as a dyad involving the older adult and the social worker. The strengths model builds upon existing resources of the individuals, their informal systems of support, and the environment and mobilizes older adults to meet expressed needs. This approach emphasizes the person-in-environment context of responses to life situations and tends to place the resolution of long-term care in a much larger arena than many traditional approaches do.

MENTAL HEALTH AND CAREGIVERS

The family is the foundation of the nation's long-term care services. Although the majority of Americans do not consider caregiving a burden, there is a cost for caring that involves many aspects of the caregiver's life. Such costs include financial costs, the effects on relationships, and emotional costs (Greenberg, Boyd, & Hale, 1992). If older adults are to avoid nursing home placements and remain in the community, policy makers and service providers must strengthen the system of support for caregivers by lessening the costs of care.

The strengths model endorses the work of informal and formal care providers by constructing collaborative efforts from the beginning. The outcome is that caregiving becomes less of a private family matter and more of a communitywide effort where cooperation is the operational term. With a focus on mental health, a strengths perspective unifies the delivery of services to older adults through a joint approach for services in preventative, acute, or chronic situations. The advantages of combining the aging and mental health systems are discussed in the following components of the strengths model.

Assessing people in their environments. Understanding the community associations a person has and building on them is crucial at any age but is especially necessary as a person ages and becomes more restricted to home. If affiliations with religious organizations, civic groups, political organizations, socialization groups, and special interest associations are recognized as sources of support by family members and formal service providers, they can become part of a matrix of nurturing and care as a person experiences crises or long-term conditions.

Collaborative assessment with other agencies. From a strengths perspective it is critical that service systems, namely the aging network and the mental health community, join forces to recognize the value of shared clients so that resources are used to prevent mental health conditions whenever possible and provide more effective intervention when necessary (Biegel, Shore, & Silverman, 1989). For this to occur there must be joint record keeping, statements of confidentiality, and eligibility requirements. The outcome would be "a series of shared experiences between workers in two systems" and an overall plan of resource planning that would benefit older adults and their families (Biegel, Shore, & Silverman, 1989, p. 161).

Building on systems' strengths. A stigma is often attached to mental health services. This is especially the case for older adults, who often do not have a frame of reference for counseling, case management, or other forms of mental health intervention. The aging network has less of a stigma and could be used as a vehicle to engage older adults with or without mental health conditions and establish communication between the populations of older adults.

Partnerships with informal support systems. The value of working with families is critical to any long-term care effort. Partnerships provide settings for mutual help or the idea that all people can be helpers as well as helpees (Rappaport, Reischl, & Zimmerman, 1992). As agencies merge and share in service responsibility, the families of older adults gain a sense that long-term care is a joint venture in which they are given the respect and attention commensurate with their roles.

PAYING FOR LONG-TERM CARE

The experiences of people receiving long-term care dramatically illustrate the serious shortcomings of a service model based on diagnosing disease and providing medical intervention. Such a model fails to adequately assist older adults with chronic conditions for which there is no quick cure. The result is unnecessarily high levels of dependency and a great loss of self-determination for older adults and their families.

If the goal of long-term care is the decrease of unwarranted dependency and the increase of assistance so that people can manage their lives despite resource and environmental constraints, a realignment of service need, funding, and available help is necessary. This can occur if the system of long-term care changes to include providing a range of nonmedical and medical services, financing services other than acute medical and institutional care, coordinating the different sources of payment for long-term care, and supporting families who provide long-term care emotionally and financially.

How can the strengths model contribute to these changes? Table 9.4 contrasts medical and strengths models of long-term care. By examining the two models it is possible to identify issues that must be addressed in the funding of long-term care.

Expanding the funding of long-term care. Approximately 90% of public expenditures for services are allocated for the health care of older adults (1987, U.S. Senate, Special Committee on Aging). The imbalance between expenditures for institutional care and those for noninstitutional care also needs to be corrected. This funding pattern results in underfunding or absence of funding in such critical areas as prevention of disease and disability, rehabilitation, and long-term care provided in an individual's home.

Coordinating funding sources. Approximately 80 different federal programs fund the programs for assistance of older persons who require long-term care (O'Shaughnessy and Price, 1987). Many of these funding resources have different eligibility requirements and coverage with specialized focuses. There is no single authority overseeing services of long-term care.

Managing preventive and long-term care systems. A medical model orientation permeates the majority of managed care systems. As a result the hospital dominates as the center of the service delivery system for long-term care. According to Bould, Sanborn, and Reif (1989) unless the hospital orientation is challenged, "many hospital-based, vertically integrated systems will not expand beyond narrow goals and services" (p. 195).

Minimizing intergenerational conflicts. Dividing services to older adults into various budgets and budgeting processes facilitates gaps in coverage and fosters failure to examine how the different needs of older adults are often inseparable from each other in life. For

TABLE 9.4　*Long-term Care: Medical Model vs. Strengths Model*

	MEDICAL MODEL	STRENGTHS MODEL
Focus of intervention	Individual	Individual, family, and communities
Focus of services	Diagnosed acute illness	Prevention of functioning decline
Goals	To cure diagnosed disease and symptoms	To support self-determination, family caregivers, and collaborative efforts
Caregivers	Trained professionals including physicians, social workers, and nurses	Family and community members with support from joint agencies
Duration of services	Short-term and long-term custodial	Continuous from private home to family residence, community and nursing home facilities
Setting of services	Hospitals and nursing homes	Individual homes, community residences, and nursing homes

example, poor housing can lead to medical problems and the subsequent need for long-term care (Callahan, 1994). Welfare and health care budgets should become integrated into a single budget with an integrated set of priorities for young and old that reflects an allocation of resources between generations and within generations.

Summary

Long-term care is as complex as the needs and wants of older adults. Although the last decades have brought progress in the scope of services, much progress needs to be made to prevent unwarranted dependency among older adults and to lessen the responsibility for families. A service continuum is needed that spans the boundaries between acute, chronic, and long-term care; health, social and mental services; and home and community settings.

A comprehensive, coordinated service of long-term care requires extending services and finances beyond the narrow limits of a medical orientation. For this reason, the strengths model offers opportunities to explore new policies and organizational structures that usher in the needed system reforms.

REFERENCES

Abel, E. K. (1989, Fall). The ambiguities of social support: Adult daughters caring for frail elderly parents. *Journal of Aging Studies, 1*(3), 211–230.

Barrow, G. M. (1992). *Aging, the individual and society*. St. Paul, MN: West Publishing Company.

Benjamin, A. E., Jr. (1985). Community-based long-term care. In C. Harington, R. J. Newcomer, & C. L. Estes (Eds.), *Long-term care of the elderly: Public policy issues* (pp. 197–211). Beverly Hills, CA: Sage Publications.

Biegel, D. D., Shore, B. K. & Silverman, M. (1989). Overcoming barriers to serving the aging/mental health client: A state initiative. *Journal of Gerontological Social Work, 13* (4/3), 147–165.

Bould, S., Sanborn, B. & Reif, L. (1989). *Eighty-five plus: The oldest old*. Belmont, CA: Wadsworth Publishing.

Brody, E. (1990). *Women in the middle: Their parent care years*. New York: Springer Publishing Co.

Callahan, D. (1994). What do we owe the elderly: Allocating social and health care resources. *Hastings Center Report, Special Supplement, 24*, (4) March-April, S3–11.

Connor, K. A. (1992). *Aging America: Issues facing an aging society*. Englewood Cliffs, NJ: Prentice Hall.

Cox, H. G. (1988). *Later life: The realities of aging*. Englewood Cliffs, NJ: Prentice-Hall.

Fogel, B. S. (1994). Psychological aspects of staying at home. *Generations*, Spring, 15–19.

Greenberg, J. S., Boyd, M. D., & Hale, J. F. (1992). *The caregiver's guide*. Chicago: Nelson-Hall.

Goffman, I. (1961). *Asylums*. Garden City, NY: Doubleday and Company.

Hashimi, J. (1988). U.S. elders with chronic mental disorder. In *North American elders: United States and Canadian perspectives* (123–139). Edited by E. Rathbone-McCuan & B. Havens. Westport, CT: Greenwood Press.

Herzog, A. R. & House, J. S. (1991). Productive activities and aging well. *Generations, 15*(1), 49–54.

Hooyman, N. R. & Lustbader, W. (1986). *Taking care: Supporting older people and their families.* New York: The Free Press.

Johnson, C. L. & Grant, L. A. (1985). *The nursing home in American society.* Baltimore, MD: Johns Hopkins University Press.

Juster, T. (1993). *Health and retirement survey,* University of Michigan. Washington, DC: National Institute on Aging.

Kane, R. L. & Kane, R. (1976). *Long-term care in six countries; Implications for the United States.* Washington, DC: U. S. Department of Health, Education and Welfare.

Lawton, M. P. (1985). The elderly in context: Perspectives from environmental psychology and gerontology. *Environment and Behavior,. 1 7*(4), 501–519.

Lawton, M. P. (1983). Environment and other determinants of well-being in older people. *Gerontologist, 23* (4), 355.

Mechanic, D. (1989). *Mental health and social policy.* Englewood Cliffs, NJ: Prentice-Hall.

Morycz, R. K. (1985). Caregiving strain and the desire to institutionalize family members with Alzheimer's disease. *Research on Aging, 7,* 329–361.

Morris, J. N. & Morris, S. A. (1994). Aging in place: The role of formal human services. *Generations,* Spring, 41–48.

Olson, L. K. (1994). *The graying of the world: Who will care for the frail elderly?* New York: The Haworth Press.

O'Shaughnessy, C. & Price, K.. (1987). Financing and delivering long-term care services for the elderly. In C. J. Evashwick & L. J. Weiss (Eds.), *Managing the continuum of care.* Rockville, MD: Aspen Publishers.

Pepper Commission, U.S. Bipartisan Commission on Comprehensive Health Care. (1990, September). *A call for action: Final report.* Washington, DC: U.S. Government Printing Office.

Rappaport, J., Reischl, T. M., & Zimmerman, M. A. (1992). Mutual help mechanisms in the empowerment of former mental patients. In D. Saleebey (Ed.), *The strengths perspective in social work* (pp. 84–97). New York: Longman.

Roff, L. L. & Atherton, C. R. (1989). *Promoting successful aging.* Chicago: Nelson-Hall.

Rowles, G. D. (1987). A place to call home. In L. L. Carstensen & B. A. Edelstein (Eds.), *Handbook of clinical gerontology.* New York: Pergamon Press.

Rubin, A. (1992). Case management. In S. M. Rose (Ed.), *Case management in social work practice* (pp. 5–20). New York: Longman.

Shadish, W. R., Silber, B. G., & Bootzin, R. R. (1984). Mental patients in nursing homes: Their characteristics and treatments. *International Journal of Partial Hospitalization, 2,* 153–163.

Shanas, E. (1979). The family as a social support system in old age. *The Gerontologist, 19,* 169–174.

Stone, R., Cafferata, G., & Sangl, J. (1987). *Caregivers of the elderly; A national profile.* Washington, DC: Dept. of Health and Human Services, U.S. Public Health Service.

U.S. Senate, Special Committee on Aging. (1985). Compilation of the Older Americans Act of 1965. Washington, DC: U.S. Government Printing Office.

CHAPTER TEN

The Emerging
Mental Health Needs
of the Baby Boomers

THE 76 MILLION AMERICANS BORN between 1946 and 1964 are the largest and longest-lived generation in the history of the United States. Referred to as the baby boomers, the generation that whimsically wondered "Will you still need me, will you still feed me, when I'm sixty-four?" (Beatles, 1967) is quickly approaching the age of bifocals. Their sheer numbers connote a need to renegotiate the social contracts between individuals, society, and government (Torres-Gil, 1992).

Throughout its history, the baby boom generation has altered life in whatever stage it entered (Dychtwald, 1989). The diaper industry prospered upon their arrival, and when the boomers began to walk, the demand for shoes and photographs significantly increased. In 1940, the baby food industry produced 270 million jars; by 1953 that number increased to 1.5 billion jars (Dychtwald & Flower, 1989). Elementary and secondary schools experienced unprecedented growth in enrollment. Specifically, between 1950 and 1960, student numbers rose from 28 million to 42 million (Russell, 1982). Correspondingly, the baby boomers generated growth in the labor force by adding more than 30 million workers between 1965 and 1980 (Russell, 1982). Along with employment came changes in consumption patterns. Baby boomers wanted houses, resulting in new highs for home construction and prices. Their homes were filled with gadgets ranging from electric can openers to entertainment centers. Beyond consumer products, the baby boom generation has supported the growth of lifelong learning, membership clubs, and day care centers. As a generation, its pace is fast, with high expectations for success and security.

Preoccupied with establishing careers, delaying childbearing, and affording a home, many baby boomers have had little time to consider aging in the context of particular social policies and services. This chapter illustrates how the strengths model addresses the challenges and opportunities of this generation in the area of mental health. The notion of building on strengths is critical for baby boomers, who will live long lives in an increasingly diverse and complex world.

The Baby Boom Generation

The baby boom generation is heterogeneous, with certain characteristics or experiences dividing the cohort into at least three distinct groups. According to Torres-Gil (1992), members of the oldest group were teenagers or young adults in the 1960s. Often considered the stereotypical baby boomer, these individuals tend to reflect the historical and sociological experiences of their time including the civil rights movement and the Vietnam War. The oldest boomers tend to be politically aware but far from the liberal or radical activists of the 1960s. It is important to remember that the majority of baby boomers were not involved in protests but rather followed the religious and political ideologies of their parents. Their politics, based on voting records, reflect more allegiance to political personalities than one political party.

In comparison, the middle group of baby boomers experienced their adolescence in the 1970s and tend to be more moderate in their social and political behavior. Caught between the turbulence associated with the oldest boomers and the consumerism connected with the youngest, the middle group tends to be traditional with respect to family structure, politics, and religion. As seen by their support and participation in team sports, civic clubs, and schools, it appears the middle boomers gravitate toward a sense of community and group causes ranging from environmental groups to school levies.

Adolescents in the 1980s, the youngest group of baby boomers, has been dubbed yuppies by the media. Described as career-oriented and materialistically focused, these boomers appear caught in a cycle of "more is better." Politically speaking, this group of baby boomers tends to be conservative and more comfortable with corporate America than the other members of their cohort.

Although the baby boomers divide into three small groups, the generation shares a sense of cohesiveness and common traits, as indicated by Figure 10.1.

As a cohort, they are not affluent, nor will the majority of boomers reach the financial security enjoyed by their parents. According to census data, only about 3.5 million have household incomes of $50,000 or more. In comparison, the income of 12.7 million averages between $18,000 and $20,000. Perhaps to their disadvantage, the baby boomers were raised during times of prosperity by parents who wanted their children to have a better life than they did. To varying degrees, their families, the media, and financial institutions encouraged the boomers to gauge one's success by one's ability to accumulate. In support of this consumption, the generation is accustomed to an economy based on credit, long-term mortgages, and deficit spending on all levels of government.

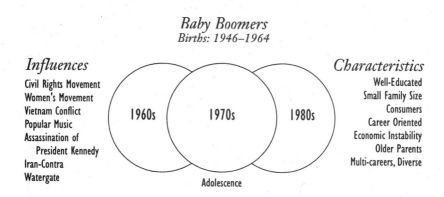

FIGURE 10.1 *Influences on and characteristics of the baby boom generation*

The group is, however, relatively well educated, with 1 in 3 having had at least some college education, which is more education than previous cohorts. Even with higher levels of education, the boomers, because of their numbers and a changing world economy, experience competition for employment, education opportunities, and social benefits, including retirement. Many have unrealistically high lifestyle expectations that place them at odds with other generations. As a result of transgenerational tensions, the baby boomers have been described as "jealous of the gold in the golden years" (Craeger, 1989, p. 16). However, the real issue has more to do with unrealistically high expectations than comparisons with previous generations.

There is an important comparison to make between baby boomers and their parents: A much larger percentage of baby boomers will be single or childless when they retire. According to Mitric (1994), 30 to 40% of the baby boomers are unmarried, compared with 20 to 25% of their parents at retirement. The rate of baby boomers remaining childless almost doubles that of their parents, which means that baby boomers are not replacing themselves. Further, those that had children had them much later in life, so baby boomers are less likely to be able to depend on a child during crisis or old age.

Another significant feature of baby boomers is that 50% of all women of this generation work outside of the home. Although they are not as likely as men to have pension incomes, millions of women boomers will be eligible for Social Security based on their own earnings. Thus, for the first time researchers are "paying attention to the wife's retirement intentions, independent of her husband's" (LaRock, 1994, p. 16). This increased financial independence, coupled with their numbers and life expectancy, places women boomers in a premiere position to advance their political power.

Diversity is an additional feature that characterizes baby boomers and adds to the generation's complexity. Though data on the lives of minorities as they age are becoming more available, it remains less than adequate. To gauge the economic status of the baby boomers as they age, one need only look at today's situation. African Americans and other baby boomer minorities remain clustered in peripheral industries that pay low wages. Consequently, in 1991 the ratio of African American family income to white income declined from 62 to 56%. In 1993, the average income of whites was $35,776 a year; the African American average was $24,856 (American Almanac, 1994). Their disadvantages derived from the economic marginality that has followed minority groups from childhood to middle age. Employment records are a central factor associated with economic security in later life. A work history that supports a good pension plan or maximum Social Security benefits is a necessary step for economic security for the baby boomers as they age.

In summary, baby boomers are advancing as primary components of America's aging nation. The political, economic, and social influence this generation will have on society remains to be seen. It is expected they will offer unique contributions to the aging process as they have throughout their life stages.

Emerging Mental Health Issues

Though it is always dangerous to forecast the future, with regard to mental health issues and baby boomers, certain predictions related to their social and economic environmental factors seem relatively safe. Since the environment is a key factor to mental health issues, certain situations will challenge baby boomers as they age. To what degree the following situations result in mental health problems depends largely on the generation's ability to share individual resourcefulness and change social policy.

Multiple Careers Changes in the economy, the demand for new products and services, and new technologies have altered the relationship workers have with particular companies. Unlike many of their parents, baby boomers cannot expect lifetime employment in a position, organization, or career. Consequently, boomers must be flexible of mind to learn new skills necessary to change their careers.

The positive outcomes of multiple careers are numerous. Baby boomers have opportunities to develop relationships with a variety of associates, establish a repertoire of skills, and design a patchwork of jobs that allow for flexible schedules. In contrast, multiple careers do not offer baby boomers the financial security and accumulation of benefits, including retirement, that previous generations enjoyed. Negotiating employment-driven transitions challenge baby boomers to find balance in their lives from sources other than employment and careers. Also, the increased competition for work and alienation from the workplace will add to life's stress unless the individuals are mentally agile and are supported by social policies that offer safeguards during interruptions in employment.

Lifelong Education Traditionally, education has been geared to prepare the young for lifetime careers. Due to the increase in multiple careers, baby boomers must begin to consider education as an ongoing, lifelong process essential for retraining in response to changes in the economy. As the need for continuous learning expands, baby boomers are expected to develop both vocationally and nonvocationally oriented interests. For example, a social worker might enroll in an art history course to complement volunteering as a docent at a local art museum.

The new imperative to view education as cyclical rather than linear confronts the myth associated with aging and loss of mental capacity and the stereotype that older people are rigid, uncreative, and unproductive. Baby boomers must chart a new course that weaves education throughout an already fast-paced lifestyle. Simultaneously, institutions of education, corporate training programs, and community-based programs must develop educational objectives that build upon the experiences of baby boomers while challenging them to stretch into diverse areas of learning.

Extended Retirement Baby boomers will probably force retirement age back to 70 years as they choose, some from necessity, some for fulfillment, to remain in the labor force (Kirkland, 1994). However, they will still experience between 10 to 20 years of retirement. Despite this recognition, a study conducted by the American Association of Retired Persons (AARP) revealed that "less than a quarter of workers over the age of forty reported that their employers were offering any kind of preretirement planning" (Moody, 1994, p. 147). The people involved in financial planning programs are usually the more educated who have funds to plan with, but the poor receive little education on Social Security or other entitlements associated with retirement.

The downward mobility of the baby boomers, caused in part by the disparity between young and old workers, high housing costs, and a standard of living beyond the realm of two paychecks, suggests economic trends are unfavorable for them to finance their future Social Security and other old age benefits. A critical question is whether Social Security should be a universal benefit or a residual insurance program involving means testing (Montgomery, Borgatta, & Kosloski, 1994). In either case, baby boomers are unable to depend on population growth to finance their future Social Security and other age benefits. The pressure of living in the present while planning for the future will only increase for baby boomers if an effective solution for financing the government and retirement benefits is not found.

Varied Family Structure Extended life and fewer children encourages baby boomers to reach beyond the nuclear family to form intergenerational relationships with friends and relatives. Transgenerational families will cause baby boomers to redefine family structures and the role of family. Whatever form the family takes, it will be severely pressured economically and socially. Baby boomers will reside alone in unprecedented numbers and more four-generation households are anticipated.

Social welfare policies must acknowledge these new relationships and provide motivations for family members to care for one another. As in the case of extended retirement, the notion of dependency in varied family structure will be a crucial aspect of public policy. One goal for baby boomers will be to develop formal and informal support systems to supplement traditional reliance on the family. Critical to these systems, transgenerational social, economic, and political relationships will provide baby boomers with the potential to replace established lines of power and obligation with a new social order.

Older People As a Resource The negative stereotypes about aging acquired in childhood tend to evolve into expectations across the life span. Boomers will have more time to confront these myths than previous generations and move society toward a new image of aging.

Included in this image will be the baby boomers' demonstrated capacity to learn, grow, and change in response to the new social and economic atmosphere. Work, volunteerism, and community service are some of the areas of opportunity that America's new aging cohort will expand to invest their accumulated knowledge and resources. Thus, whether it is through environmental causes or supporting school levies, the baby boom generation will have a special role in affecting the quality of life in their communities.

As Americans age but maintain their health and increase their level of activity in the work force and community, obstacles that could prevent older people from full participation in life will be confronted. Thus, baby boomers are expected to engage in life activities differently from generations of the past and in such a way as to complement rather than conflict with generations of the future.

Diversity in Aging The baby boom generation reflects the diversity of American society. An issue to address is the nation's ability and willingness to equitably accommodate the 8 million immigrants who came to America during the 1980s (Moody, 1994). This influx of people, most of whom are Asian or Hispanic, represents a figure comparable to the number who came to America in the early 1900s. Though the majority of immigrants are young, their aging will make the baby boom generation far more diverse than generations of the past.

Similar to minority groups, the role of gender needs consideration because cumulative disadvantages negatively influence retirement financing. Divorce, employment ceilings, child care responsibilities, and widowhood have a disproportionate effect on women. The different realities of men, women, whites, and minorities will dictate reforms in Social Security, long-term care, income security, and other social welfare policies. Baby boomers must consider the unresolved issues of basic rights and entitlements to reduce the threat of conflict and address the varieties of aging experiences.

Poverty Lack of income is a major concern for baby boomers. Approximately 9 million boomers currently live in poverty, a number that is expected to accelerate with age. The gap between the rich and poor is likely to widen as the earning power of the affluent increases while the poor remain entrenched in problems associated with the underclass, including unemployment, illiteracy, and substandard housing. Further, the structural changes in social institutions, such as the economy, have left people with little hope of competing in the job market of the 1990s and beyond.

Traditional social insurance and public assistance programs are inadequate shields against poverty. The baby boomers must form a consensus about the best methods to address poverty by exploring their values, beliefs, and attitudes related to human needs and obligations of society.

Applying the Model to the Baby Boom Generation

The personal and social environmental factors facing baby boomers influence their ability to engage in an array of relationships with success and potentially threaten their mental health. For example, inadequate income is an antecedent of social stress often resulting in depression, anxiety, and alienation. However, the question is not of what mental health problems the baby boomers might experience but rather of how the problems can be prevented or addressed before causing disruptions in the rhythm of life.

The strengths model creates a new agenda for social work by placing personal and social empowerment at the core of practice. Personal empowerment encourages people to take direction in the helping process and to learn new patterns of thought and behavior in relation to unique life situations. Social empowerment recognizes that people's "definitions and characteristics cannot be separated from their context" (Cowger, 1994). People with social empowerment have the resources and opportunities to play a significant interactive role in shaping the environment.

As interdependent dynamics, personal and social empowerment are significant for the baby boom generation as it reallocates resources and seizes opportunities to reshape the environment to address the demands of the approaching century. Promoting empowerment through strengths places baby boomers in a position of power consciousness, whereby their numbers become less of a threat to other generations and more of a positive force capable of promoting social and economic justice through revised social policy. Thus, the strengths model considers empowerment as a useful tool in collaborative efforts to achieve equitable distribution of societal resources.

Placing the strengths model in the context of the baby boom generation is important for several reasons. First, it moves the model from a clinical focus to one of prevention, demonstrating the model's versatility and commitment to changing the balance of power among individuals and social structures. Second, the strengths model supports achieving social justice between generations by collaborative assessments in dynamic environments. This aspect is essential for baby boomers faced with generational conflicts unless the present system of paying for benefits and entitlements is substantially altered. Finally, the strengths model discovers uniqueness in individuals and environments. Given the unique qualities of the baby boomers, the model provides a structure for matching generational uniqueness with interventions to create an environment compatible with needs. This quality of the strengths model as well as its components are discussed below.

Persons and Environment

Figure 10.2 illustrates major environmental influences on the baby boom generation. Though all aspects of the environment have an impact on the boomers, it is the economic forces that present the biggest challenge. Attempts to advance on career ladders, establish financial security, accumulate assets, and plan for retirement will take more personal energy and perseverance for baby boomers than previous generations. For the poor of this generation, the chance to confront the obstacles of poverty will decrease as the gap between the rich and poor widens.

The downward economic mobility of baby boomers provides a backdrop against which their longevity must be measured. If the tendency is that the generation will live longer and have fewer assets, the question becomes, "Who will care for the baby boomers as they age?"

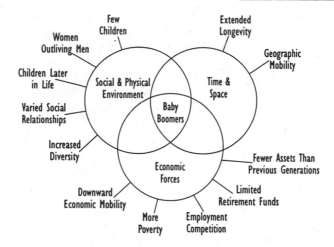

FIGURE 10.2 *Persons, environment, and the baby boom generation*

In considering their social environments, the answer is not children or even extended family members. Rather, the boom generation must create new forms of caregiving and lifestyles for the last stage of the life cycle.

Ideally, the strength of the boomers' environment is its diversity. Besides racial and ethnic differences, the baby boom generation can expect various family structures and social relationships to emerge. As the boomers age, women will outlive men on the average of 7 years. This will influence new concepts for the role of women, especially in relation to caregiving and work in the competitive job market. Thus, diversity will usher dramatic changes in the political landscape, affecting not only older people but the entire society. It will prevent the baby boomers from becoming complacent and stagnated by bringing to the forefront competing demands, disparate interests, and vocal interest groups.

COLLABORATIVE ASSESSMENT

When conducted with an individual, a collaborative assessment presents a holistic perspective of a person by defining individual strengths in life situations. The relationship between the client and practitioner is critical to collaborative assessment because it positively influences dialogue and mutual trust.

Collaborative assessment as a component of a strengths perspective of prevention involves understanding collective power as a strategy to achieve personal and political goals. A number of factors affect collaborative assessment in this context:

- Values and beliefs concerning power
- Attitudes related to the distribution of resources
- Perceptions of diversity
- Self-interests versus interests of the group
- Political dimensions

In social work practice based on strengths, with the "client" being not an individual but rather a group of people representing a generation, collaborative assessment occurs on the macro level with political institutions and social welfare organizations. Assessment extends beyond individual concerns to the broader environment depicted in Figure 10.2 and involves a process of consciousness raising, critical thinking, and action (Cox & Parsons, 1994). The primary difference between this process and the action of interest groups is that egalitarian relationships or partnerships result from collaborative assessment rather than relationships of dominance.

Collaborative assessment entails recognizing and building on strengths. Table 10.1 illustrates these aspects of the baby boom generation.

Individual Strengths

Certain themes emerge from the list of strengths associated with the baby boomers. One is they generally have a flexible mindset in reference to career changes, geographic residences, and education. Much of this flexibility reflects survival techniques and strategies to preserve mental health in a changing economy; however, the fact remains that change is a part of their lives.

Another theme of the generation is its diversity. As a strength, diversity will affect social welfare programs, the distribution of resources, and the financing of benefits (Torres-Gil, 1992). However, the overriding theme of strength is the baby boomers' longevity. They will

TABLE 10.1 *The Baby Boom Generation:*
A Strengths Perspective

STRENGTHS OF BABY BOOMERS	POSSIBLE INFLUENCE
Longevity	Restructuring of senior citizen benefits
	Revision of health care policy
	Advances in medical technology and research
	Long-term political activity
	Demands for leisure
	Altered view of work and retirement
	New role for women
Mobility	Restructuring of state and local governments
	Expansive informal and normal systems support
	Disproportionate numbers of people in geographic regions
Diversity	Restructuring of social policies
	New roles for members of racial and ethnic groups
	Culturally or ethnically based long-term care
	Recognition of an assortment of languages, food, and customs
Well educated	Understanding of political and economic systems
	Familiarity with social service systems
	Career options

have more time than any other cohort to exert political influence, without creating conflict between generations, by enhancing the interconnectedness of life from infancy to old age through social policies and programs.

Formal and Informal Supports

Figure 10.3 describes the formal and informal support systems of the baby boom generation. In terms of formal support, the baby boomers are more familiar with social services than previous generations, namely the array of counseling options. This is because the growth of mental health services corresponds to the growth of baby boomers, beginning with services to veterans when the majority of baby boomers were born, to the 1963 Community Mental Health Act when they were adolescents and young adults. Memberships clubs, including fitness centers and housing communities, are anticipated to offer baby boomers socialization support. Other forms of support offered by member organizations might be home deliveries, medical hotlines, buying clubs, and travel opportunities.

Transgenerational support is expected to be a significant source of informal support for baby boomers. Longevity and altered traditional family structures, namely fewer children, fewer couples, and more people alone, will encourage baby boomers to extend across generations to form relationships. Though these relationships will result in ethical and power issues, the hope is baby boomers will dissolve the boundaries that separate generations and develop new lines of communication and obligations.

GENERATIONAL PROGRAM PLAN

A program plan for the baby boom generation overlaps the wants of individuals, small groups, and the generation as a whole. Table 10.2

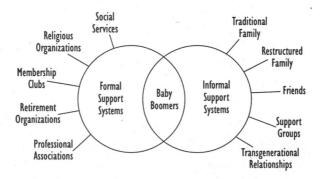

FIGURE 10.3 *The formal and informal support systems of baby boomers*

TABLE 10.2 *Baby Boomers: A Program Plan*

	WANTS	STRATEGIES

MICRO: Individual	Personal freedom
	Security
	Financial opportunities
	Leisure options
	Health care
		State wants and limits
		Explore thoughts on
		  growing old
		Engaging in lifelong
		  education
		Learn about retirement,
		  health, housing,
		  recreation options

MEZZO: Small Groups	Recognition of varied
	  family structures
	Sense of community
	Cross-cultural group
	  preparation
		Develop support networks
		Advocate family policy
		Form mutual aid groups
		Explore cultural/gender/
		  ethnic stereotypes

MACRO: The Generation	Reduced transgener-
	  ational conflict
	Equity in distribution of
	  resources
	Participatory government
	Redefinition of aging
	Redefinition of work and
	  retirement
		Design new programs
		Engage in political activity
		Organize groups across
		  generations
		Change social policy

defines these wants and corresponding strategies on three levels, with corresponding strategies for action.

The wants of baby boomers on all three levels reflect the crucial importance of their attitude and relationship toward younger groups. Baby boomers must accept social responsibility for themselves in terms of health care and retirement, while proactively addressing the wants of minorities, the poor, and children. Transgenerational is a watchword that runs throughout the generation's program plan.

Another feature of the program plan is the importance placed on political activity. The changes baby boomers make on a personal or micro level will have a direct impact on the political scenario for the generation as a whole. For example, as individuals assess their health and retirement plans, collective impetus for change on a broad-base level is likely to grow. The interconnectedness of individual baby boomers with the entire generation is viewed as a strength, and the well-articulated wants of individuals are likely to change the way government does business and how society views older people.

EVALUATION

Evaluation necessitates a review of how successful the generation's wants are met. Guidelines for evaluation include:

1. Do the changes distribute resources in an equitable manner across generations?

2. Are the issues of entitlements, rights, and public assistance resolved for the good of society?

3. Are individuals empowered to initiate change in their lives that improves the quality of life?

4. Does the action lessen the gap between the rich and poor?

5. Has the view of older people been revised to reflect older people as a resource for the nation?

6. Does action prevent environmental factors associated with issues of mental health, including depression and anxiety?

The evaluation process related to baby boomers and the prevention of problems in mental health assesses the relationships within levels of intervention, individuals, small groups, and generations. It is assumed that there is a mutual influence across levels, so that individual change does make a difference in the large picture and the process of accumulated change takes place over time.

Summary

This chapter examined how the strengths model can be used as a tool for preventing mental health problems in the baby boom generation. It suggested that the boom generation has particular strengths that have the potential to change environmental conditions that negatively affect the ability and capacity to cope constructively and achieve some control over life during the aging process.

Influencing the environment requires a sense of power. This means that baby boomers as individuals and as a generation must assess and use their strengths to exert power with a world view by questioning social policies and examining transgenerational relationships. Thus, the strengths model encourages baby boomers not merely to live a long life but to use life experiences to enrich society.

REFERENCES

The Beatles. (1967). When I'm sixty-four. *Sergeant Pepper's Lonely Hearts Club Band*. London: Apple Records.

Cowger, C. D. (1994). Assessing client strengths: Clinical assessment for client empowerment. *Social Work, 39*(3), 262–268.

Cox, E. O. & Parsons, R. J. (1994). *Empowerment-oriented social work practice with the elderly*. Pacific Grove, CA: Brooks/Cole.

Craeger, E. (1989, June 20). Baby boomers are jealous of the gold in golden years. *Detroit Free Press*, p. 14.

Dychtwald, K. & Flower, J. (1989). *Age wave: The challenges and opportunities of an aging America*. Los Angles: Jeremy P. Tarcher.

Kirkland, R. I. (1994, February 21). Why we will live longer and what it will mean. *Fortune Magazine*, pp. 66–77.

LaRock, S. (1994). Boom(er) or bust?, *Aging Today, 15*(4), 7, 10.

Mitric, J. M. (1994). Baby boomers not yet ready for prime time. *Aging Today, 15*(3), 1–2.

Moody, H. R. (1994). *Aging: Concepts and controversies*. Thousand Oaks, CA: Pine Forge Press.

Montgomery, R. J. V., Borgatta, E. P., & Kosloski, K. D. (1994). Social policy toward the older worker. In H. R. Moody (Ed.), *Aging: Concepts and controversies* (pp. 320–336). Thousand Oaks, CA: Pine Forge Press.

Russell, L. (1982). *The baby boom generation and the economy*. Washington, DC: The Brookings Institute.

Torres-Gil, F. M. (1992). *The new aging*. New York: Auburn House.

U. S. Bureau of the Census (1994). *American almanac: Statistical abstract of the United States*. Texas: The Austin Press.

Index